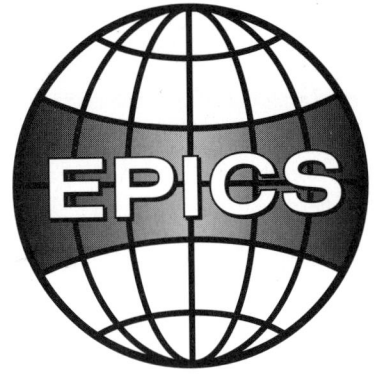

OF HEALTH AND WELFARE

Michael Witherick

Series Editor
Michael Witherick

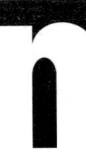

Text © Michael Witherick 2002

Original illustrations © Nelson Thornes Ltd 2002

The right of Michael Witherick to be identified as author of this work has been asserted by him in accordance with the Copyright, Designs and Patents Act 1988.

All rights reserved. No part of this publication may be reproduced or transmitted in any form or by any means, electronic or mechanical, including photocopy, recording or any information storage and retrieval system, without permission in writing from the publisher or under licence from the Copyright Licensing Agency Limited, of 90 Tottenham Court Road, London W1T 4LP.

Any person who commits any unauthorised act in relation to this publication may be liable to criminal prosecution and civil claims for damages.

Published in 2002 by:
Nelson Thornes Ltd
Delta Place
27 Bath Road
CHELTENHAM
GL53 7TH
United Kingdom

02 03 04 05 06 / 10 9 8 7 6 5 4 3 2 1

A catalogue record for this book is available from the British Library

ISBN 0 7487 6731 2

Page make-up and illustrations by Multiplex Techniques Ltd

Printed and bound in Great Britain by Ashford Colour Press

Acknowledgements
The authors and publishers are grateful to the following for permission to reproduce photographs and other copyright material in this book:

Arnold, *Human Geography: a Welfare Approach* (1977) – fig. 6.3; Blackwell, *Geographies of Health* (2001) – figs 3.6, 3.10, 5.7, 5.8; Philip's *Modern School Atlas* (93rd edition) – figs. 4.2, 4.3, 6.7; Routledge & Kegan Paul, *Health, Disease and Society* (1987) – figs 1.4, 2.3; *The Times* – figs 2.7 (11/1/02, some additional info supplied by WHO), 3.11 (11/8/01), 6.9 (12/1/02), 6.10 (21/5/01, some additional info supplied by HMSO).

Associated Press – fig. 7.9; Jorgen Schytte/Still Pictures – fig. 4.8; TDR (Special Programme for Research and Training in Tropical Diseases) – figs 3.3, 3.5, 5.7, 7.8; WHO – figs 5.6, 7.3.
Corel 638 (NT) – cover image.

The publishers apologise to anyone whose rights have been inadvertently overlooked and will be happy to rectify any errors or omissions.

Contents

1 Welfare in focus — 4
  A The nature of welfare — 4
  B The questions of welfare geography — 6
  C Measures and indicators — 7
  D Welfare and development — 13
  E The concept of human security — 15

2 The world of disease — 17
  A A diagnosis of diseases — 17
  B Diseases of age and affluence — 19
  C Infectious diseases and epidemics — 24

3 The spread of disease — 29
  A The role of the natural environment — 30
  B The human hand — 36
  C Modes of transmission — 38
  D The HIV/AIDS pandemic — 39

4 The burden of disease — 44
  A Demographic impacts — 44
  B Migration — 47
  C Wider consequences — 49
  D Repercussions of the AIDS pandemic — 51

5 Healthcare provision — 53
  A Different modes — 53
  B National strategies — 54
  C International providers — 57
  D Grass-roots initiatives — 61
  E So who gets what, where and how? — 65

6 A wider view of welfare — 68
  A The environmental dimension — 68
  B The economic dimension — 72
  C The social dimension — 76
  D Multiple deprivation and its vicious circles — 81
  E Meeting needs — 83
  F Ways forward — 84

7 Future threats and challenges — 88
  A Diseases old and new — 89
  B Global warming — 92
  C Valuing people — 94
  D Paying for welfare — 97
  E Reducing welfare disparities — 100

Further reading and resources — 104

CHAPTER 1

Welfare in focus

SECTION A

The nature of welfare

Most English dictionaries show that there are three different meanings given to the word **welfare**:

- financial and other aid given to those in need
- success and prosperity
- health and well-being.

The first of these definitions is the one most commonly implied in everyday usage, as for example in the terms **welfare state** and **welfare work**. Both are about providing help in the form of **welfare services**, such as housing, healthcare, schooling and employment.

The **welfare state** is a nation geared to provide the best possible minimum standards of living, health, housing and education. Very much in focus here are the poorer members of the population, who are unable to reach those standards by themselves. Immediately following the Second World War (1939–1945), the UK became a welfare state. Markers included the setting up of the National Health Service (NHS), the provision of free education for all and the introduction of state pensions. Since then, there has been a steady weakening of the utopian fervour that marked the early postwar years. Signs of this include developments such as private hospitals and private medical insurance, personal pension schemes, student loans to meet university fees and so on. Some would argue that the welfare state still exists in the UK, in that it remains targeted at the least prosperous members of our society, but only as a safety net. However, the inadequacy of the state pension for an increasingly elderly population, and the gradual withdrawal of state help for the unemployed and single-parent families (to name but two groups in need), do not seem to square with the idea that the welfare state in the UK is in good shape.

In some countries, such as the USA and Canada, people are expected to fend much more for themselves. But even there, the term **being on welfare** is heard. It signals the basic fact that, even in affluent societies, there are members who are incapable of providing for their own welfare and who need to be helped. Equally, there are many more countries where there is distinctly less welfare provision, as for example amongst the ranks of less economically developed countries (LEDCs). In some, it reaches the point of being almost non-existent. In contrast, one of the diagnostic features of socialist countries, such as China, Cuba and the former Soviet Union, is the centralised provision for all citizens of most of those things recognised as the key components of a welfare state.

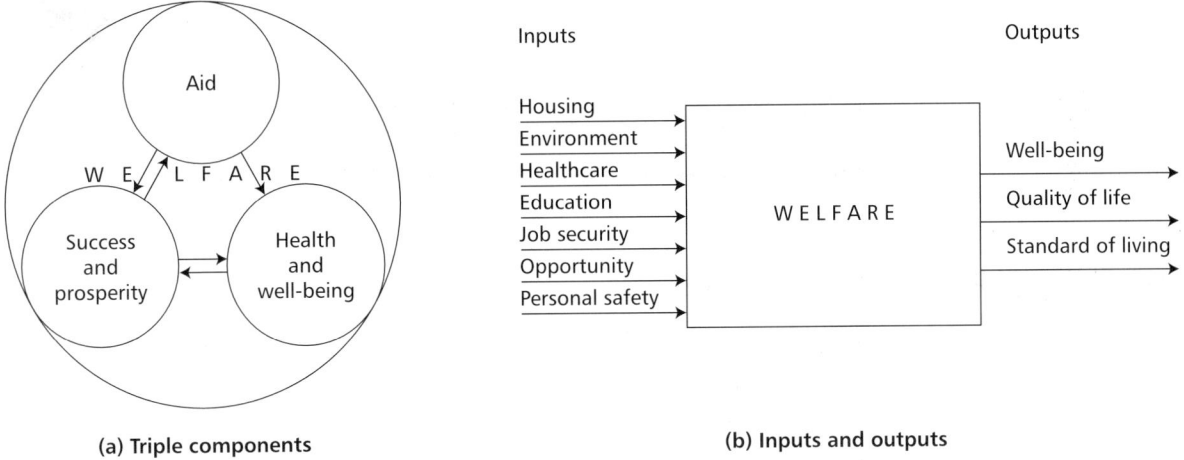

(a) Triple components (b) Inputs and outputs

Figure 1.1 Two views of welfare

The links between welfare as 'aid' and the other two definitions given at the very beginning are shown in **1.1a**. Success and prosperity allow the nation–state to invest in the good of its citizens. At an individual level, they give people choice and a better guarantee of a comfortable and secure lifestyle. The third definition might be seen as more of an outcome, in that welfare means the promotion of better health, housing, education and a whole host of other things that are largely to do with **well-being** and **quality of life**. These two terms are regularly encountered in welfare studies. They are often used interchangeably, so we can perhaps assume – in this book at least – that they virtually mean the same thing. They refer to the general condition of a person or population produced by the interaction of a wide range of factors such as are shown in **1.2**.

Welfare as discussed in this book will be mainly about providing for the **needs** of people. This includes not only the provision of **services** (housing, schools, healthcare, water supply, transport and so on) but also the creation of **opportunities** (to work, to feed, to enjoy life, to realise ambitions and so on). Ensuring the **access** of people (particularly the needy) to those services and opportunities is a vital part of welfare. These services and

Figure 1.2 Some components of quality of life (well-being)

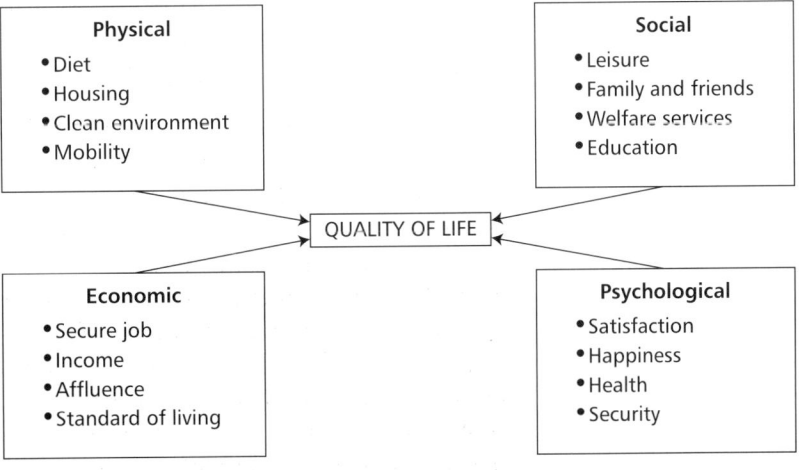

WELFARE IN FOCUS   5

opportunities may be seen as the **inputs** to a **welfare system** (**1.1b**). The system **outputs** are those conditions that are variously described as well-being, quality of life and sometimes **standard of living**.

> ### Review
>
> 1 Who pays for the welfare state?
>
> 2 Explain the links between the three components shown in **1.1a**.
>
> 3 Check that you understand what is meant by a **system**, and what might be involved in a **systems approach** to welfare.

SECTION B

The questions of welfare geography

Welfare geography is an approach to human geography that was born in the 1970s and that persists to this day. It focuses on issues such as unemployment, homelessness, poverty, crime, access to education, healthcare and other social services. The geographer's particular interest in welfare centres on spatial variations in

- the **need** for
- the **provision** of
- and **access** to

those things that we have just identified as welfare inputs (**1.1b**). The fact of the matter is that there are huge and often abrupt spatial variations in welfare, be it globally, regionally or locally.

It has been said that welfare geography is about 'who gets what, where and how' (**1.3**).

- The '*who*' refers to the different components of a population (that is, its subdivision into ethnic groups, socio-economic classes, age cohorts and so on). Implied here is the idea that not all groups within a population necessarily have equal access to welfare provision.
- The '*what*' is about that provision, and therefore all those things that impact on human happiness and well-being (specifically, the inputs shown in **1.1b** and **1.2**).

Figure 1.3 The main directions of welfare geography

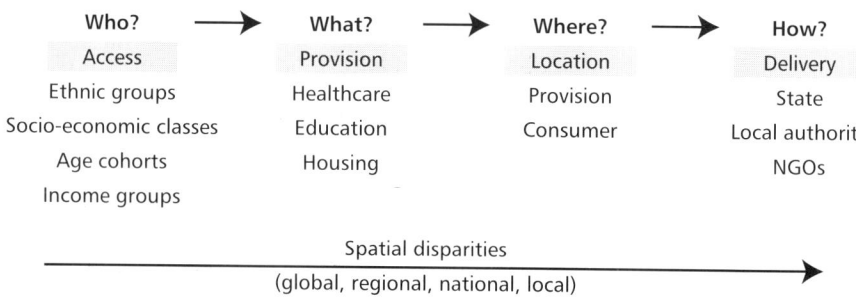

- The *'where'* has two aspects, namely where services are located and where people, as consumers of those services, happen to live. The coincidence of those two things can profoundly affect the quality of life.
- The *'how'* is about the processes that deliver welfare (its services and opportunities) within society. In particular, it brings into focus those institutions that manage or control that delivery. These might be the state, the local authority, non-government organisations (NGOs) such as the charities and aid agencies, or private companies.

Underlying all four questions of welfare geography is the theme of spatial inequality or disparity (**1.3**). The painful fact today, as throughout history, is that the inputs and outputs of welfare (**1.1b**) are not evenly distributed across the face of the Earth. There is a huge and widening gulf (known as the **development gap**) between the quality of life enjoyed in the rich more economically developed countries (MEDCs) and the poorer LEDCs. But even within each of these two 'worlds', there are striking national differences, as for example between the UK and the Ukraine, or Mexico and Ethiopia. Narrowing the spatial focus still further, we realise that within individual countries strong contrasts exist at a local level, particularly between different groups of people.

In short, welfare geography recognises the existence of different states of welfare around the globe. Those differences prevail both between and within nations.

Review

4 Put together your own definition of **welfare geography**.

5 Focusing particularly on housing, community amenities, social services and environmental quality, identify examples of welfare disparities within your home area.

SECTION C

Measures and indicators

Given this focus on welfare's variations from place to place, a vital need in any geographical study must be to find some sound indicators of their existence. Ideally, what we want are measures that will allow us to show those variations in map form. It goes without saying that any assessment of welfare is going to involve more than one measure. After all, we have already made the point that welfare is a many-sided thing. Figures **1.1b** and **1.2** indicate the major dimensions of welfare, so we might use these as guidelines in our search for suitable measures.

Health

Good health is something that we all hope for. Without it, daily living is drained of much of its enjoyment. For this reason alone, health is the most emphasised single dimension of welfare. In geographical studies, it has two distinct but related facets:

- the incidence of disease
- the provision of healthcare.

With the former, the relationship to welfare is an inverse one. A high incidence of disease implies a low level of welfare. With the latter, the relationship is a direct one. Good healthcare provision contributes significantly to welfare.

When it comes to mapping the incidence of disease, there are many (too many) to choose from. The World Health Organization (WHO), an agency of the United Nations, collects vast amounts of data on the global incidence of a wide range of diseases. This is particularly true for **infectious** or **communicable diseases.** These are either passed on by physical contact between people or are transmitted by animal and insects, known as **vectors**. The diseases include malaria, cholera, typhoid, smallpox and polio. They are most prevalent in the countries of the Tropics, with their high rates of fertility and youthful populations (**1.4a**). Also in this group is today's number one, worldwide scourge – HIV/AIDS.

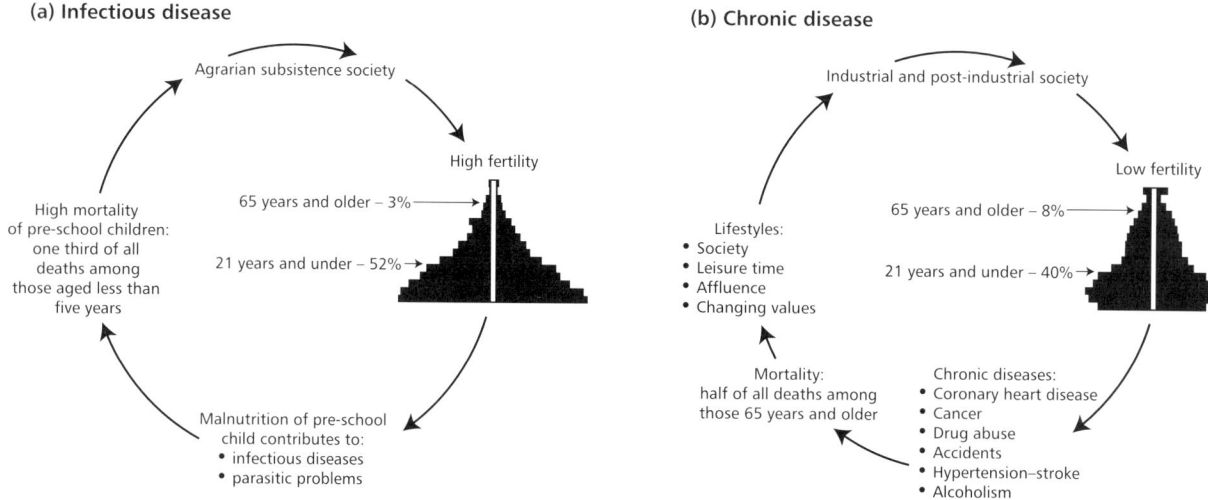

Figure 1.4 Models of two different disease scenarios

Non-infectious diseases are a diverse group, but they include the **chronic degenerative diseases** associated with:

- ageing (such as cancer, arthritis and dementia)
- lifestyles and living conditions (strokes, respiratory complaints and heart disease; **1.4b**).

In general, these diseases are more associated with the MEDCs.

Case study: Standardised mortality rates

Medical researchers and geographers frequently want to compare the mortality rates of different places. In doing so, however, they need to allow for the fact that one area might have an older population than another. Older people are more likely to die than the young, so the age structure of an area's population needs to be taken into account. This is done by comparing the age structure of the area with that of the country as a whole. This then allows researchers to calculate the death rate that would have been expected had the area's age structure been identical to that of the nation as a whole. An index value of 100 indicates that the death rate of a particular area is the same as for the country as a whole. A value greater than 100 indicates that the death rate of the area is higher than might be expected given its age structure.

The incidence of disease is known as **morbidity**. This is not to be confused with **mortality** – the incidence of death. We should also remember that, whilst spatial patterns of mortality may provide some sort of summary picture of the fatal victims of morbidity, there are other contributors to death. Accidents and deaths during pregnancy and birth are just such. Equally, it is important to recognise that the killer nature of a disease can be increased if the person who contracts it happens to be in poor general health. This might be the result of malnutrition or a lack of prior exposure and immunity. Indeed, with poor health normally 'non-serious' illnesses, such as German measles and gastro-enteritis (inflammation of the lining of the stomach and intestines), can quickly become killers.

Healthcare is rather more difficult to measure, because its quality and accessibility are as important as its quantity. However, the most commonly used measures, such as the number of people per doctor or nurse, the number of hospital beds and the percentage of GNP spent on health, assess quantity rather than quality (**1.5**). They tell us little about accessibility.

Figure 1.5 Some indicators of welfare in a sample of countries (1995)

HDI ranking	HDI value	Doctors per 100 000 people	Primary school enrolment (% of age group)	Daily calorie intake	People without access to safe water (%)	People below income poverty line (%)	CO_2 emissions per capita (tonnes)
High							
Japan	0.924	177	99	2905	1		10.5
UK	0.918	164	92	3237	1	13	9.5
Uruguay	0.826	309	94	2830	5	25	1.8
Medium							
Mexico	0.786	107	99	3137	15	34	3.7
China	0.701	115	99	2844	33	11	2.8
Kenya	0.519	15	65	1971	47	37	0.3
Low							
Laos	0.491	32	73	2143	56	46	0.1
Bangladesh	0.440	18	75	2105	5	48	0.2
Ethiopia	0.298	4	35	1845	75	est. 85	0.1

> **Review**
>
> 6 What are the advantages of using standardised mortality rates?
>
> 7 Check that you understand the difference between:
> - **morbidity** and **mortality**
> - **infectious** and **non-infectious** disease
> - **chronic** and **curable** disease.
>
> 8 If you do not know about the Human Development Index (HDI) as referred to in **1.5**, be sure to read the **Composite measures** subsection below.

Education

Few would doubt that education provides the doorway to those positive outcomes of welfare that we might sum up as 'a better future'. Education sets in motion a virtuous upward spiral. It increases awareness of opportunities and the ability to exploit them; and it increases the chances of finding work. Thus education provides access to those things that many people would define as being central to well-being and a good quality of life, such as a well-equipped house, leisure time and a safe environment. The United Nations Development Programme (UNDP) uses a range of measures, such as **enrolment ratios** (percentages of relevant age groups) at the primary, secondary and tertiary levels of education (**1.5**). The **adult literacy rate** is another obvious measure, as is expenditure on education as a percentage of GNP.

> **Review**
>
> 9 Sketch a diagram to show the virtuous upward spiral that you think is created by education.

Food security and diet

Having enough food to eat today and being sure that the same will apply tomorrow is the most basic of all human concerns. Food is the very means of life. Lack of food is the very essence of poverty – it has been described as 'the ultimate exclusion'. For these reasons, it is perhaps the most fundamental aspect of welfare. Food security has a direct bearing on health. Too little food leads to malnutrition, which in turn increases vulnerability to disease and reduces the ability to work. Starvation lurks in more extreme circumstances and can lead directly to death. Perhaps the most widely used measure in this context is daily calorie intake (**1.5**), but it is more an indicator of today's food consumption rather than any certainty about tomorrow's meals.

> **Review**
>
> 10 Suggest a definition of **food security** and give reasons why it may be difficult to measure.

Housing

Literally having a roof over one's head is a very basic need of people the world over. This is particularly the case in those parts where some sort of protection from the elements (for example, from cold and heavy rain) is

> **Review**
>
> 11 Can you think of any other ways of assessing the housing aspect of welfare?

vital in the interests of survival and personal comfort. One might argue that the need for housing is directly proportional to the inclemency of climate, and for that reason the need varies globally. Where substantial shelter is required for most if not all of the year, good indicators of the housing situation include the level of homelessness and the percentage of the population with or without access to safe water and sanitation (**1.5**). The amount of dwelling space per capita might also serve as an appropriate measure.

Employment

In most parts of the world, access to the three basic human needs of food, shelter and clothing is secured through having work. You either provide for yourself, as is the case with the so-called subsistence farmer or, as a factory hand or office worker, you earn money to purchase these basic wants. The incidence of long-term unemployment is certainly a telling measure here, as also income per capita. The latter needs to be assessed on a national basis and related to what each country defines as its **income poverty line** (**1.5**).

> **Review**
>
> 12 Find out what is currently defined as the income poverty line in the UK.

Environment

There are two distinct aspects here:

- the state of the physical environment in which the individual lives and works, the central issue here being one of pollution
- the nature of the social environment, which embraces such things as crime and personal safety, freedom of speech, ethnic harmony, equal opportunities and leisure.

A wide range of measures exists to assess the degree to which the physical environment is degraded and polluted (**1.5**). The situation is rather different, however, as regards the social environment. Obvious indicators are perhaps provided by crime and female activity rates. In MEDCs, where leisure is an important part of everyday life, perhaps the average number of hours worked each week might be a useful indicator.

> **Review**
>
> 13 Name four measures that are widely used to assess environmental quality.
>
> 14 Identify those factors that you think contribute to a person feeling socially excluded or isolated.

Composite measures

Given that welfare is a many sided condition (**1.1b** & **1.2**), it follows that measurements confined to a single aspect, such as those considered so far, are going to be of limited value. Multivariate measures, which touch on as many of the different facets as possible, are better. To this end, the UNDP now regularly uses one such measure to assess the stark welfare contrasts that exist around the world and to monitor change. It is known as the **Human Development Index** (**HDI**).

The HDI was devised in 1990 and takes into account three variables: income per capita, adult literacy along with the percentage of children attending school, and life expectancy. Thus it touches on the employment, education and health dimensions of welfare. The HDI value can range from 0 to 1 (from worst to best). The wealthiest of the MEDCs score index values approaching 0.999 and the poorest countries range down to less than 0.300. The most recent Human Development Reports now classify countries into three groups: high human development (HDI values 0.800 and above); medium human development (0.500–0.799) and low human development (less than 0.500) (**1.5** & **1.6**).

The HDI has a number of advantages:

- it is easy to understand
- it relies on data that are generally available throughout the world in a reasonably reliable and up-to-date form
- it provides a basis for ranking all the countries of the world
- it allows assessments to be made of the progress that countries make over time.

Its main drawback is that its scope is limited to only three aspects of welfare.

The UNDP has also devised other multivariate measures, such as the **Gender-related Development Index** (**GDI**) and the **Human Poverty Index** (**HPI**). The first is important in that it recognises that the status of women in today's society is a vital input to welfare. The latter attempts to assess welfare more in terms of poverty and deprivation. Both indices take into account more variables than the HDI, but require more sophisticated data. Such data are simply not available for many of those countries where gender inequality and poverty are major issues.

Figure 1.6 The global pattern of human development

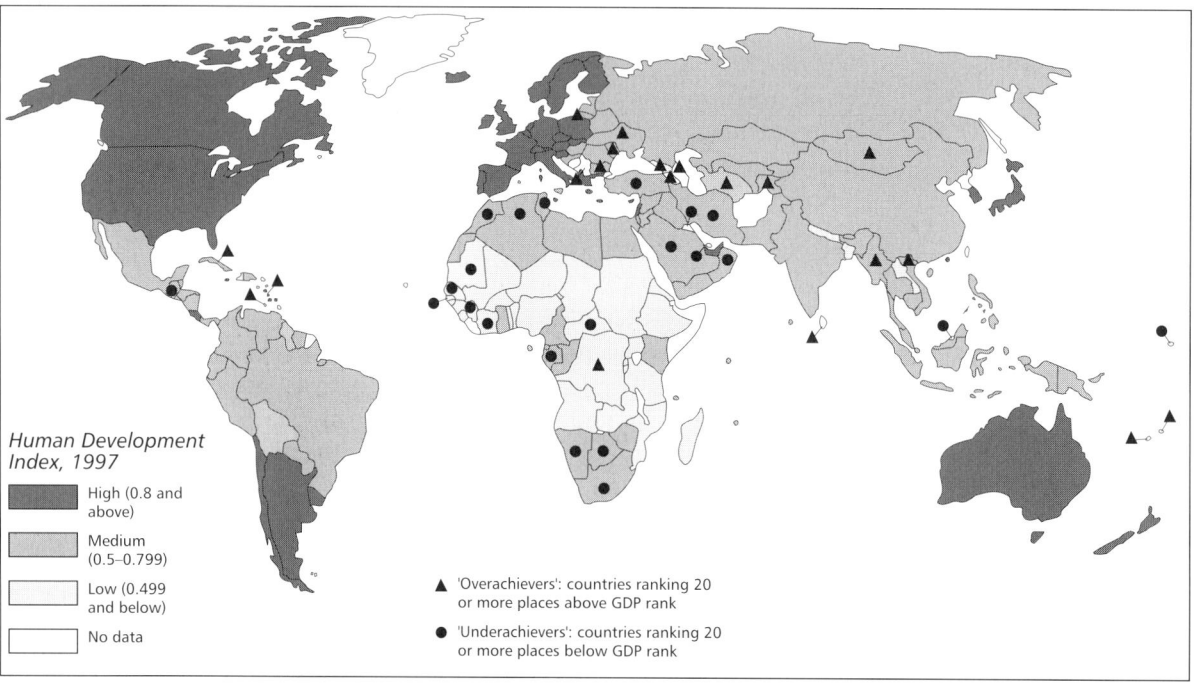

> **Review**
>
> 15 What conclusions do you draw from the data in **1.5**?
>
> 16 Summarise the main features of the distribution pattern shown in **1.6**.
>
> 17 Suggest reasons why gender equality is an important aspect of welfare.
>
> 18 Why might it be better to assess welfare in negative terms, such as deprivation and poverty?

SECTION D — Welfare and development

In the previous section, the term **development** began to enter the discussion. It is important that we have a clear understanding of the term and its relationship with welfare.

Although there is no universally agreed definition of development, most would agree that it shows the following characteristics:

- it is a process of change that operates over time
- it is essentially positive in character, in the sense of bringing benefits
- it involves exploiting resources (physical and human) and moving towards a more advanced state
- its precise character and speed vary from place to place and over time, creating differences between and within countries
- it is a complex process and, like welfare, involves many different strands.

The debate in geography and other disciplines about development is to do with the relative importance of those different strands. On the one hand, it is argued that economic growth is the powerhouse, or driving force, of development. The wealth created by economic growth drives progress in all the other strands. In contrast, there are those who believe that development is about satisfying basic human needs, achieving greater social justice and improving the quality of life (**1.1b**).

Development has been likened to an electrical cable (**1.7**). Through it passes the power by which countries and societies progress from primitive to more advanced states. The core of the cable is made up of an 'alloy' of economic growth, technology and enterprise. The power flowing through this core comes largely from the exploitation of natural and human resources. At any one time, the amount of energy flowing along the cable depends on two factors: the rate and scale of resource exploitation, and the cable's carrying capacity. Pulses of acceleration and deceleration in the rate of development result from changes in these two factors.

Around the core, but an integral part of the cable, is a 'casing' woven from many different strands. Whilst the general specification of the cable is basically the same the world over, its 'wattage', or carrying capacity, can vary from place to place, and from time to time. A high-capacity cable allows more power to pass through and can therefore support faster development. Cutting the cable at any point along its length will reveal a cross-section. The collective condition of the components thus exposed represents what is known as the **level** (**stage** or **state**) **of development**.

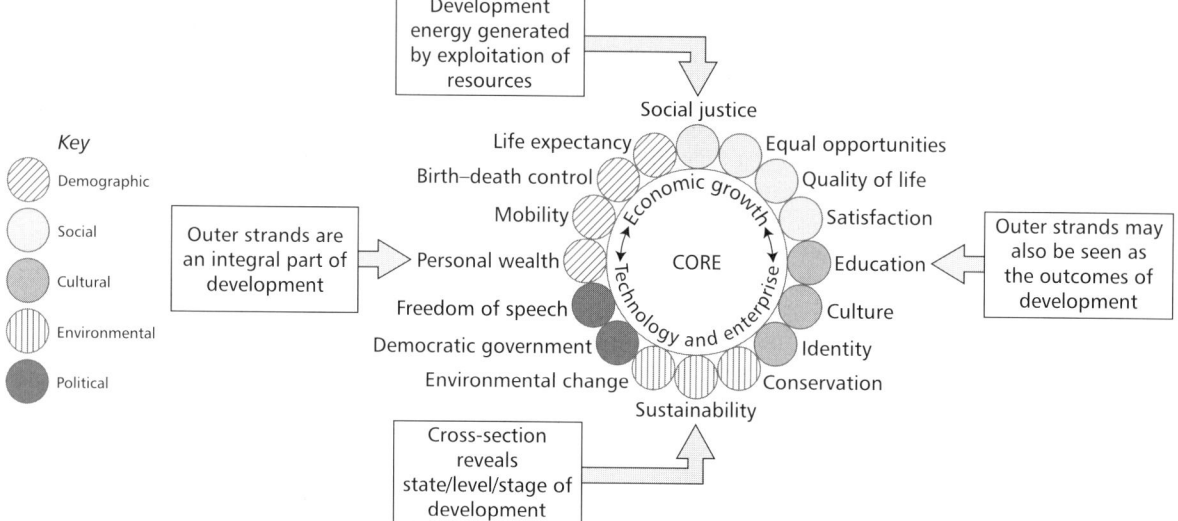

Figure 1.7 The development cable

It is when we look at the outer casing of the cable that the link between development and welfare becomes apparent. Welfare is largely that casing; it is a collection of the outcomes of most of those outer strands. You will see that the main components identified in the key to **1.7** coincide roughly with the main facets of welfare discussed in the previous section. In short, welfare is a vital part of development: it is also the major collective outcome of the process.

In medical geography, reference is increasingly being made to the **disease** (or **epidemiological**) **transition**. This concerns changes in the pattern of disease now being experienced in LDCs that are related to the development process. The five changes involved in the transition are:

- a rise in chronic degenerative diseases, associated with falling birth and death rates and the rapid ageing of populations
- an increasing incidence of non-communicable diseases (such as cancer, heart disease and diabetes), linked to changes in lifestyle
- the pandemic of HIV infection and AIDS
- a rise in the burden on healthcare systems resulting from the previous changes
- a rise in mortality from accidents and suicides in young adults.

When it comes to establishing the degree of relationship between welfare and development, the easiest way is to take a measure of each. Life expectancy and per capita income are widely recognised as two fairly reliable summary indicators of welfare and development, respectively. It is left to you to test the

Review

19 In your own words, explain what is meant by **development**.

20 Can you think of any other outer strands that might be added to **1.7**?

21 Can you explain the five changes of the **disease** (or epidemiological) transition?

relationship between these two measures for yourself as an Enquiry exercise (guidance is provided in the box at the end of the chapter).

Looking at the relationship between development and welfare over time and at a national level, we may say that, in general, development is a force for the good. It raises levels of welfare. Figure **1.4** illustrates that in the context of disease and health. But the benefits of improved welfare are rarely equally shared by all the citizens of a country. All too often, there is a widening gap between rich and poor, between the 'haves' and the 'have nots'. Pockets of deprivation are increasingly apparent in a general landscape of rising prosperity. The same principle applies at a global level. Economic globalisation is widening the gap between MEDCs and LEDCs, creating a landscape with considerable variations in levels of welfare (**1.5**). Thus today's world of welfare is counter-directional: progress and deprivation exist side-by-side.

SECTION E

The concept of human security

The UNDP has introduced the concept of **human security** (**1.8**). This is based on the idea that development in its fullest sense (that is, **human development**) leads to a widening of people's choices. Human security is the condition that allows people to exercise these choices safely and freely. It is woven from seven strands, and may be seen as being safe from chronic threats such the hunger, disease and repression that, unhappily, remain a part of everyday life for far too many people.

Human security also has to do with sustainability and confidence in the future. In other words, it needs to be achieved in a sustainable way, and protected from sudden or damaging disruption. Such disruption might range from natural hazards to epidemics, from pollution to ethnic conflicts, or from the collapse of businesses to acts of international terrorism. Sadly, we live in an age of global insecurity that threatens everyone's sense of well-being. The horrendous events of 11 September 2001 were a stark reminder of this. Ironically, advancing globalisation seems to diminish, rather than promote, global security.

To sum up, welfare is a condition that is woven from a number of different strands (**1.8**). Of these, health is often singled out as being particularly crucial. The idea of human security is also important, whether it is with respect to food, work, housing, the environment or our place in society. Welfare is an integral part of, and the most telling outcome of, development. No less significant is the fact that welfare varies in the two dimensions of space and time. The former is of particular interest to us in the remainder of this book. Throughout, however, we should remember that welfare is not just about today. It is also about securing a better tomorrow.

Figure 1.8 The strands of human security (UNDP)

Category	Examples
Economic	Regular, properly rewarded employment
Food	Enough food to eat; a balanced diet
Health	Freedom from disease; access to healthcare
Personal	Human rights; educational opportunities
Environmental	Safe water and air; respect for biodiversity
Cultural	A sense of belonging; freedom from discrimination
Political	Democratic government; freedom from oppression

Review

22 Explain what is meant by the statement that 'human security is a two-sided condition'.

23 Can you think of any other events that might disrupt human security?

24 Re-read this chapter and make a definitive list of welfare's different strands.

Enquiry

1 This is an exercise to investigate the relationship between welfare and development.

   a Select a sample of countries (say, 30 overall) to represent each of the three HDI groupings (**1.5**).
   b Collect data about life expectancy and per capita GNP for your sample of countries.
   c Graph the data.
   d What conclusions can you draw from your graph?

   (A useful data source for this exercise is the annual Human Development Report produced by UNDP. The exercise may be extended to investigate the relationship between other measures.)

2 Whilst it is the responsibility of all governments to ensure that the welfare needs of all their citizens are met, a number of international organisations have been set up to assist where help is needed. Research two of the following organisations:

- Food and Agriculture Organization (FAO)
- Organization for Economic Cooperation and Development (OECD)
- United Nations Children's Fund (UNICEF)
- United Nations Development Programme (UNDP)
- United Nations Educational, Scientific and Cultural Organization (UNESCO)
- World Bank
- World Health Organization (WHO).

   a For each, find out:
   - when it was established
   - its particular aims and activities
   - its member countries.

   b What are the essential differences between your chosen organisations?

CHAPTER 2

The world of disease

It is widely recognised that health is the single most important strand in the make-up of **welfare**. Health tends to be viewed in two contrasting lights. The 'gloomy' side is about the incidence of illness and disease; the focus is on morbidity and mortality (**2.1**). The 'bright' side is about healthcare and positive moves being made in the global struggle against disease and ill health. Clearly, these two aspects are closely related, if only in a basic 'demand and supply' sense. To put it crudely, poor health creates the need for more and better healthcare. Would that the link was this simple! The relationship is complicated by a whole range of factors. Perhaps the most telling of these is the cruel fact that so often the need for healthcare is greatest in those parts of the world that are least able to provide and deliver it. It would be no exaggeration to call this one of the great global disparities.

SECTION A

A diagnosis of diseases

Today, something like 1800 different diseases are recognised worldwide – many are potentially fatal. The number is overwhelming, so how are we to begin to understand their general character and behaviour? A useful first step is to reduce the number of diseases to manageable proportions, and to do this by grouping them into categories, such as have been used in the plotting of **2.1**.

In the previous chapter, two broad types of disease were distinguished: **infectious** (sometimes called **communicable**) **diseases** and **degenerative diseases**. The latter are largely associated with the ageing of the human body. They are often described as **chronic**, in that they are typically deep-seated or long-lasting. Another word used here is **acute**. **Acute diseases** are those – such as heart attacks, strokes and appendicitis – that start abruptly, last perhaps only a few days and then either settle or develop into chronic conditions that lead to death.

Another basic distinction is often drawn between endogenic and exogenic diseases. **Endogenic diseases** are those linked to a person's make-up; you might say to their genes. Examples include most forms of cancer, circulatory (heart) and respiratory (breathing) diseases (**2.1**), as well as degenerative conditions such as multiple sclerosis, and Alzheimer's and Parkinson's diseases. In contrast, **exogenic diseases** are linked in some way to environmental conditions in the broadest sense. Such conditions range

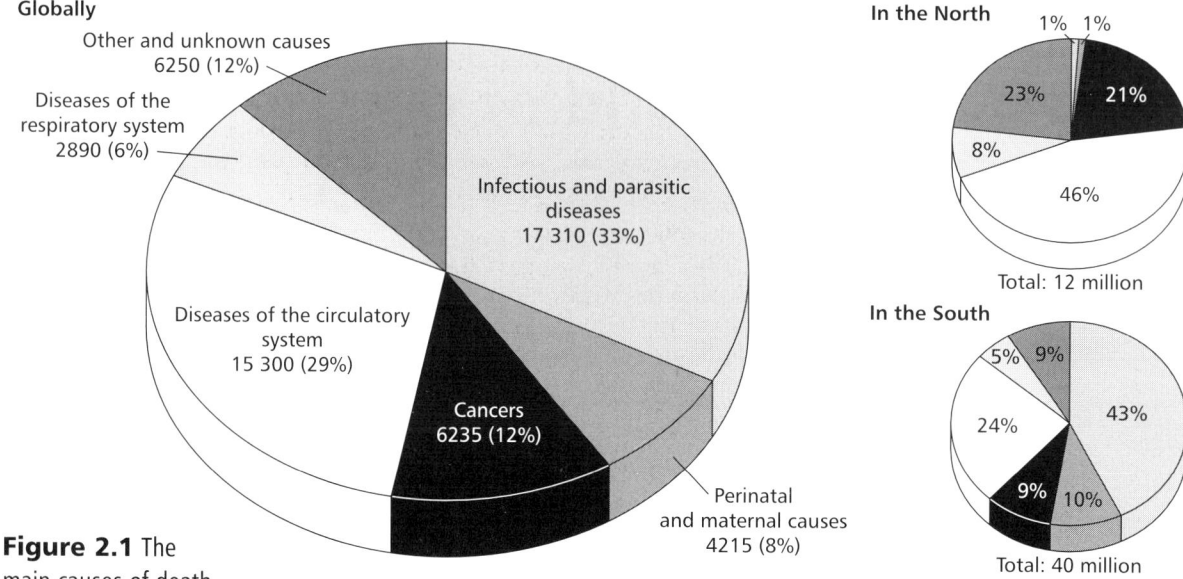

Figure 2.1 The main causes of death

Review

1 Distinguish between **endogenic** and **exogenic** diseases.

2 In which category do you think the following diseases fall:
 - diabetes
 - epilepsy
 - influenza
 - measles
 - rheumatism
 - whooping cough?

3 Refer to **2.1**. How do the North and South differ in terms of the causes of death?

from climate and housing to lifestyles and behaviour. Typical diseases include today's big killers such as HIV/AIDS, TB and malaria, along with 'less serious' diseases, such as bronchitis, and 'less common' diseases such as silicosis.

The distinction between endogenic and exogenic is not always clear-cut. For example, there are diseases, largely of a non-infectious kind, whose causes are by no means certain. Whilst cancer generally is recognised as falling in the endogenic category, it is now established, for example, that smoking is a major factor in lung cancer. That suggests that we should perhaps put lung cancer in the exogenic category. However, not all smokers develop lung cancer, and not all lung-cancer sufferers are smokers. A similarly clouded situation exists with respect to heart disease. It is regarded as an endogenic disease, but eating habits are now identified as a major contributory factor. What we need to grasp is that whilst people may be genetically disposed to certain diseases, the actual development of the conditions can be triggered by exogenic or behavioural factors such as smoking, drinking and poor diet.

Of course, it is possible to classify diseases in a number of other ways, as for example according to:

- their morbidity, particularly where they occur and their frequency of occurrence within different populations
- their 'seriousness' – in other words, their likelihood of proving fatal.

SECTION B

Diseases of age and affluence

In this section, the geographical spotlight is very much on the North. The diseases to be discussed are the main 'killers' in the MEDCs (**2.1**). There is an ironic situation here. Modern medicine and healthcare have extended life expectancy. In the UK it has almost doubled over the last 150 years. But in so doing, they have also changed the rankings in the North's killer league table. Some, like bubonic plague and smallpox, dropped out of the table altogether some time ago; whilst others, such as cancer, heart and respiratory diseases, have gained promotion. So whilst one set of killers has faded away, another set has come into the frame. Those that have faded away were largely exogenic (environmental). They were to do with the unhealthy living conditions (insanitary housing, poor diet, pollution and so on) that once prevailed in the UK and other MEDCs. In contrast, the 'newcomers' are largely degenerative in character. They are associated with the inevitable wearing out over time of both the human body and the mind. They are essentially the diseases of ageing. The brutal fact of the matter is that we all have to die. Accidents and suicide apart, some illness or disease will eventually get the better of us! Every death has a cause.

Most of the 'new killers' share two other characteristics. First, they are non-infectious. Secondly, although they may be classified as endogenic, they are also increasingly recognised as being connected in some way with modern lifestyles, behaviour and the so-called 'age of affluence'. For example, it is now well established that a greatly increased incidence of heart disease is related to the fact that we in the North are eating too much, particularly of those things (fats, sugar and meat) that are potentially damaging to health. In short, there are exogenic factors at work. Modern living, particularly its pace and stress, is also playing a part in promoting a range of ills, from alcoholism and drug abuse to mental illness and suicide.

Finally, and we hardly need reminding, there is one new killer quite unlike the rest. This is HIV/AIDS – a convenient shorthand for the **human immuno-deficiency virus** and **acquired immuno-deficiency disease syndrome** – with the former leading to the latter. Here in the North, it has not yet reached the top rankings in the killer league table, but it is highly infectious and readily spread by intravenous drug-taking and today's more liberal attitudes towards sex. We will look in more detail at AIDS in the next section and again in the next two chapters. For the moment, let us focus on two case studies involving diseases that are currently hitting the headlines in the UK.

Case study: Eat, drink and smoke, for tomorrow we die

The map of heart disease shows one of the most striking divisions between the South and the North of the UK (**2.2a**). Heart disease is encouraged by poor diet, excessive drinking and smoking. These are

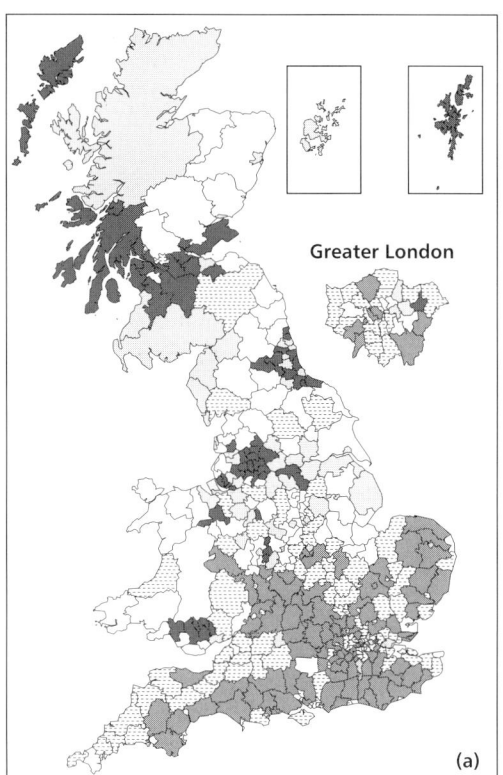
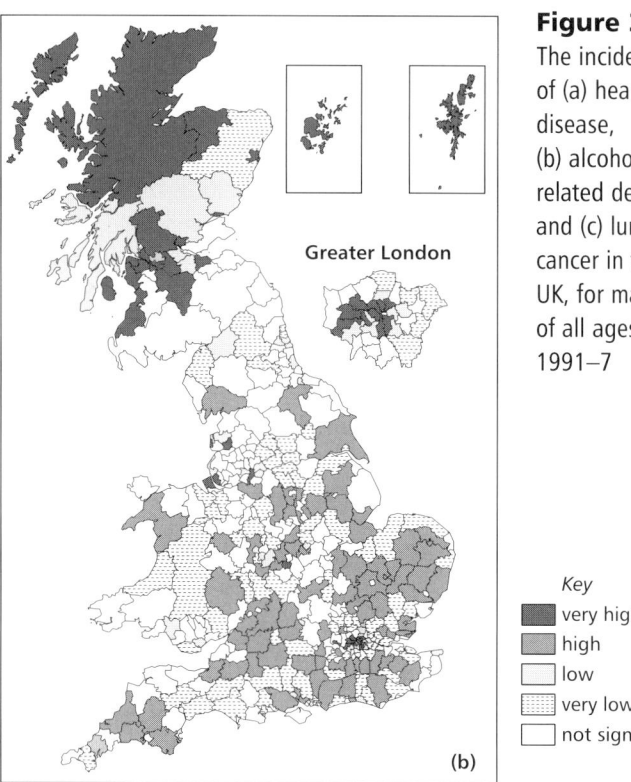

Figure 2.2 The incidence of (a) heart disease, (b) alcohol-related deaths and (c) lung cancer in the UK, for males of all ages, 1991–7

Key
- very high
- high
- low
- very low
- not significant

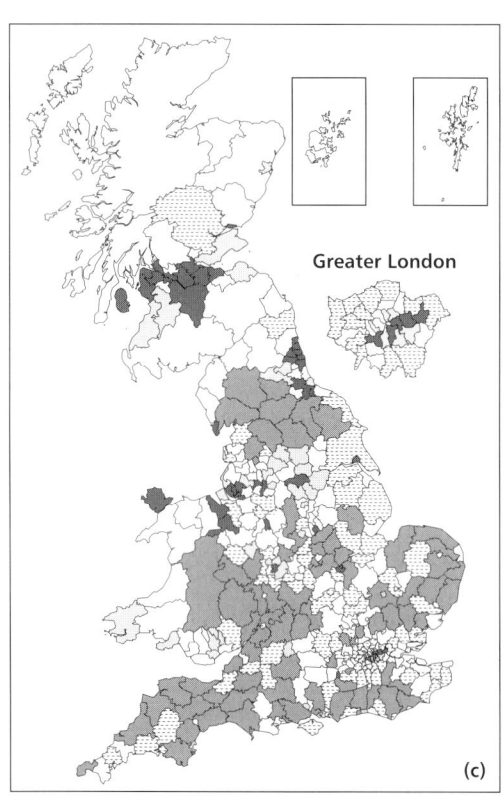

worse in South Wales, in the urban areas of northern England and over much of Scotland. The spatial pattern is very much the same for both men and women.

Food-wise, the nub of the problem is as follows:

- We are eating too much – this leads to obesity and unnecessary strain on the heart.
- We are eating too much of the wrong things (dairy products, meat and sugar) – these tend to clog the blood circulation system. Statistics show that we are eating much less by way of fresh fruit, vegetables and cereals, and we are now paying the cost.

Excessive consumption of alcohol greatly increases the likelihood of high blood pressure, cancer and cirrhosis of the liver. Alcohol abuse claims more lives in Scotland than in any other part of the UK. The death rate from alcohol-related illness in Scotland is twice that south of the border (**2.2b**). Although the overall level of drinking is not much higher in Scotland, binge drinking is more common.

Almost all lung cancer is linked with smoking, a habit that is most common among manual socio-economic groups and in the industrialised areas of central Scotland and northern England. Figure **2.2c** shows the lung cancer map for men; again, that for women is almost identical. Regional differences in smoking account for much of the north–south health divide in the UK, since smoking also increases the risk of heart disease and stroke. Despite decades of health education, the creation of smoking-free public areas and moves to discriminate against smokers when it comes to insurance and access to healthcare, recent years have seen a levelling off in the general decline in smoking. A quarter of the population aged 16 and over still smokes. Notions that smoking is in some way 'cool' or is good for stress and slimming are seriously misplaced.

So, smokers, drinkers and unhealthy eaters be warned!

Figure **2.2** clearly illustrates the fact that disease has a spatial dimension; its occurrence varies from place to place. Geographers are primarily interested in the distribution pattern (that is, morbidity). Having identified that pattern, however, the next step is to try to explain it. This is where we can get into difficulties, particularly if we try to see matters in too simple cause-and-effect terms. We know instinctively that there may be environmental factors, such as pollution, climate and water supply, to be taken into account. Equally, we are aware that occupation and social class can play a part. For example, there are occupational diseases, such as silicosis associated with mining, and there is a higher rate of fatal accidents amongst manual workers. We also recognise the significance of a person's genetic make-up.

You may have noticed that in the last case study, the word 'cause' was not used, even where we know that there is a strong link between smoking and lung cancer. In seeking explanations, medical geographers and epidemiologists prefer to adopt a concept known as **multiple causality**. In a nutshell, this recognises the complexity of the real world. Each effect is seen as having a number of causes, and each cause as producing a number of effects (**2.3**). This is something that needs to be understood. It was implicit in our earlier discussion of the possible connection between smoking and lung cancer. It is spelt out more clearly in the next case study and in **2.5**.

Figure 2.3 Multiple causality

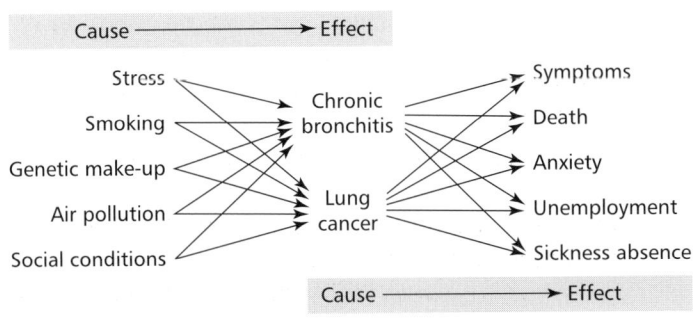

Case study: 'Breast cancer toll tops smoking deaths'

This was the recent headline in a British newspaper following a report by two major cancer charities late in 2001. Breast cancer is now the most common form of life-threatening cancer in the UK. With an estimated 39 500 cases diagnosed each year, the disease has narrowly overtaken lung cancer, with an estimated 38 900 cases. Skin cancer is more common than either, with 44 000 new cases a year, but it is seldom fatal. Whilst lung cancer rates are higher amongst men, breast cancer is almost, but not completely, the preserve of women.

Figure 2.4 The incidence of breast cancer in the UK, for females of all ages, 1991–3

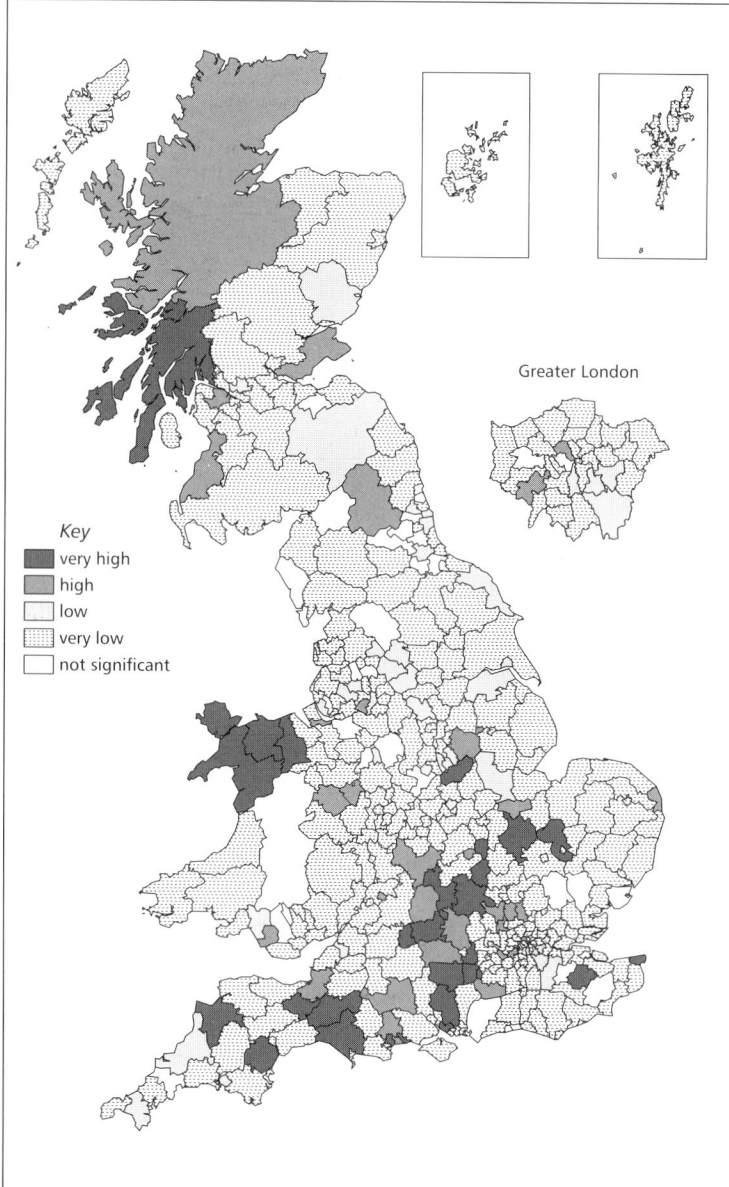

The reasons for the steady rise in breast cancer over the past 30 years are unclear. Certainly, mass screening programmes have played a part in raising the number of diagnosed cases. By improving personal awareness of the symptoms of the disease, better health education has increased detection. Breast cancer is age-related, and since women are living even longer, it is hardly surprising that its incidence is on the rise. But a number of lifestyle factors may also be contributing to the upward trend. For example, more women are choosing to have children later in life and this is now thought to increase the chances of developing the disease. This might explain the high incidence in the affluent areas of south and central England, where there are relatively large numbers of career women (**2.4**). The high rates in North Wales and the north-west of Scotland are more perplexing. Obesity in post-menopausal women is thought to be a risk factor, but is the situation any different in these high-rates areas compared with the rest of Wales and Scotland? As with most forms of cancer, the genetic factor is important, but perhaps there are others of which we are as yet unaware. There could be a link with environmental pollution, or with food. Who knows?

THE WORLD OF DISEASE

The best general barometer of the success or otherwise of a population's life-long fight against disease and death is life expectancy. Whilst life expectancy throughout the UK showed impressive gains during the 20th century, spatial differences show little or no signs of diminishing. For example, a recent ONS survey showed that men in Dorset live 10 years longer than men in Glasgow. It would seem that places can damage your health and survival. Equally, there are places that are good for your health and survival. The answer to why people in one part of the country live longer and apparently healthier lives than those in another part is multi-causal. Most likely it is to do with the character of places, some crucial aspects of which are set out in **2.5**. It may also be to do with the type of people who choose to live in those areas of longevity.

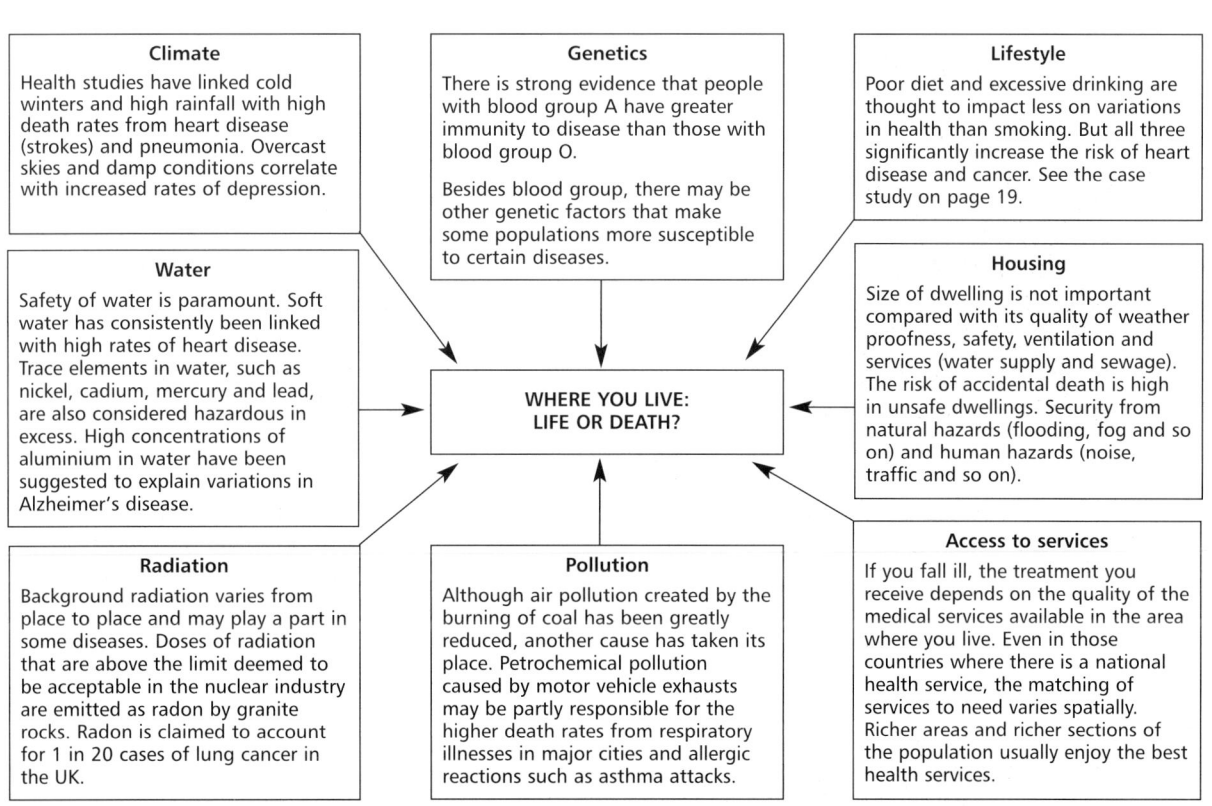

Figure 2.5 Factors affecting life expectancy

Review

4 Write an explanatory account of one of the maps in **2.2**.

5 Draw a multi-causal diagram like **2.3** that would apply to the case study of breast cancer.

6 Figure **2.5** is a model based on the situation in an MEDC. What changes, if any, would you make to it so that it is valid for the situation in an LEDC? Give your reasons.

SECTION C

Infectious diseases and epidemics

The previous section should lead to the conclusion that, globally, one of the main health challenges in the North is dealing with chronic degenerative disease and changing lifestyle habits. Is the challenge the same in the South? The short answer is 'no', because here it is the infectious diseases that are the main killers (**2.1**). These diseases tend to fluctuate over space and time, with sporadic and serious outbreaks developing into **epidemics**, followed by periods of quiescence. The only similarity with the North is that changing traditional lifestyle habits can play a part in checking the spread of these diseases. The most serious infectious diseases in today's LEDCs are shown in **2.6**. But remember two things:

- a number of these diseases once prevailed in the MEDCs, but they have been completely eradicated there
- some of the diseases still occur in MEDCs, but they are perhaps better contained and treated, and so made less life-threatening.

Disease	Symptoms and prognosis	Associated factors
AIDS (HIV)	HIV removes resistance to opportunistic infections and so prepares the way for AIDS. Weight loss, diarrhoea and swollen glands. Six-year incubation period. It is estimated that more than 40 million people are HIV-positive. Incurable.	Transmitted by sexual contact, contaminated saliva, blood and hypodermic needles. No particular environmental conditions, but most prevalent in urban areas.
Cholera	Symptoms develop suddenly after an incubation period of 1–5 days. Severe vomiting and diarrhoea, which can quickly lead to dehydration and death.	Associated with poor sanitation and where safe drinking water is scarce.
Dengue fever	Occurs in four forms. Most commonly causes painful joints, fever and rash; in the fatal haemorrhagic form, there is bleeding from the mouth and nose. Some 2.5 billion people are at risk. No vaccine; no specific treatment; no cross-immunity between the four forms.	Transmitted by mosquito. Poorly drained areas in the Tropics and subtropics.
Diarrhoeal diseases	Can range from mild diarrhoea and vomiting to acute dehydration. Probably affect the greatest number of people worldwide, but usually not fatally. Curable by antibiotics.	Transmitted by touch and by contaminated food and water. No particular environmental conditions.
Malaria	Fever possibly leading to liver/kidney failure and heart/lung complications. 270 million people affected. Incurable, but preventive drugs available.	Transmitted by mosquito. Poorly drained areas in the Tropics and subtropics.
Measles	Severe catarrh, spots inside mouth, rash. Epidemics every 2–3 years. Mostly children affected; about 1 million deaths. Vaccine available, but may not provide lifelong protection.	Spread by infected people coughing and sneezing. No particular environmental conditions.

Disease	Symptoms and prognosis	Associated factors
Polio	Affects central nervous system and can lead to paralysis. Estimated 10 million physically handicapped survivors. Effective vaccine available.	The virus is excreted in faeces, so the disease is most common in areas of poor sanitation.
Sleeping sickness	General debilitation. 140 million people affected. Few effective drugs.	Transmitted by tsetse fly. Most prevalent in humid tropical areas.
Typhoid	High fever, rash and possible inflammation of spleen and bones. 16 million cases a year. No long-lasting vaccine.	Transmitted through contaminated food and water.
Tuberculosis	Fever, weight loss, spitting blood. Nine million new cases each year. Was curable with antibiotics.	Spread by coughing and sneezing. Bad housing, poor diet, unhealthy environment.
Yellow fever	Aching muscles, headache and fever; can attack kidneys and heart. Reduced mortality due to immunisation.	Transmitted by mosquito. Tropical rainforests of Africa and South America.

Figure 2.6 Infectious diseases that are prevalent in the South

The following case studies take a look at two infectious diseases. One of them, typhoid, has been around for a long time and was once quite widespread in the North. The other is dengue fever, a relative newcomer. Like typhoid, it particularly afflicts people in the South. Examination of two of the 'big killers' (malaria and HIV/AIDS) must wait until the next chapter.

Case study: Tracking down typhoid

Perhaps one of the most famous victims of typhoid was Prince Albert, the husband of Queen Victoria, who died of the disease in 1861. At one time, it was a major killer in Europe. It was normally associated with overcrowding, poor sanitation, defective sewers and inadequate washing facilities. A fractured and overflowing sewer at Windsor was the culprit in Prince Albert's case. However, the slum conditions that favoured the disease had largely disappeared in Britain by the 1930s.

There are about 100 cases of typhoid in the UK each year. At the time of writing, the last outbreak was at Newport (South Wales) in August 2001. In the overwhelming majority of British cases today, the infection was caught overseas. Infections are diagnosed in this country most often during the summer months when drains and beaches abroad become smellier. Contrary to popular belief, the Mediterranean region is not free of typhoid.

Typhoid is spread only by human beings. The bacterial organism is carried in faeces and urine, and is usually spread to food by either flies or unwashed hands. The incubation period is between 10 and 14 days. If not diagnosed and treated in the first two weeks following incubation, all manner of complications can set in. It is these complications – such as pneumonia, meningitis and intestinal haemorrhage – that kill.

Although typhoid may be largely banished from the UK, worldwide there are reckoned to be 16 million cases of typhoid fever a year and more than 600 000 deaths. Eighty per cent of these are in Asia and most of the others in Africa and Latin America.

One particularly worrying aspect of typhoid is the existence of **chronic carriers**. These are people who have contracted the disease. Although they recover, they continue to carry the disease in their faeces and urine for months, even years. So long as they do so, they can transmit it to others. It is estimated that around 40 per cent of chronic carriers respond to a long-term course of antibiotics. Unfortunately, the bacterium responsible for causing the disease has developed a resistance to commonly used antibiotics. Thus it is becoming increasingly necessary to treat carriers with either 'heavier' medicinal therapies or even surgery (removing the gall bladder, in which the disease lingers). But so long as a single chronic carrier remains untreated, so typhoid will persist.

Case study: Dengue fever on the rampage

Dengue is a vector disease, carried by a particular species of mosquito known as *Aedes aegypti*. It is the female that is the carrier. She must feed on blood in order to reproduce. Biting one human after another to obtain that supply of blood often results in the mosquito transmitting the disease from an infected to a non-infected person. Exactly the same principle applies to the spread of malaria and yellow fever, except that different species of mosquito are involved.

Dengue fever is a viral infection and four main types are recognised. The mildest type causes influenza-like symptoms – painful joints, fever and an irritating rash. There is no specific treatment: in this form the disease usually runs its course in a week. This form is rarely fatal, but patients need lengthy convalescence. The haemorrhagic type cases the victim to bleed from the mouth and nose, to suffer excessive thirst and to have difficulty breathing. There is no cure, and so mortality can be quite high.

One of the particular problems with dengue fever is that there is no cross-immunity. Contracting one type of dengue fever does not give immunity to the other three. Moreover, the haemorrhagic type seems to occur most often in people who have already been exposed to one of the other types.

The disease is widespread throughout much of Asia and Latin America, with over 100 million cases reported each year. Factors contributing to the increased incidence of dengue fever include:

- rapid urbanisation
- population movement
- the resistance of the vector mosquito to insecticide
- the inadequate provision of piped water.

At present, the prognosis is not encouraging. There is little that can be done to check the spread of the disease.

We can perhaps draw some comfort from the fact that during the 20th century medical science mounted a number of highly successful campaigns against often fatal infectious diseases. These included measles, polio, diphtheria and whooping cough. A disease not shown in **2.6**, smallpox, has been completely eradicated. To date, this is the only global infectious disease to be eliminated. As late as the mid-1960s, smallpox was endemic in 31 countries (it flourished in Britain up to the 19th century), and between 10 and 15 million people were stricken each year. Of these, some 2 million died, and millions of survivors were left blinded or badly disfigured by its pitted scars. At the end of the 1960s, a global campaign involving the vaccination of over 250 million people led to the eventual disappearance of the disease. The last reported case was in Somalia in 1979.

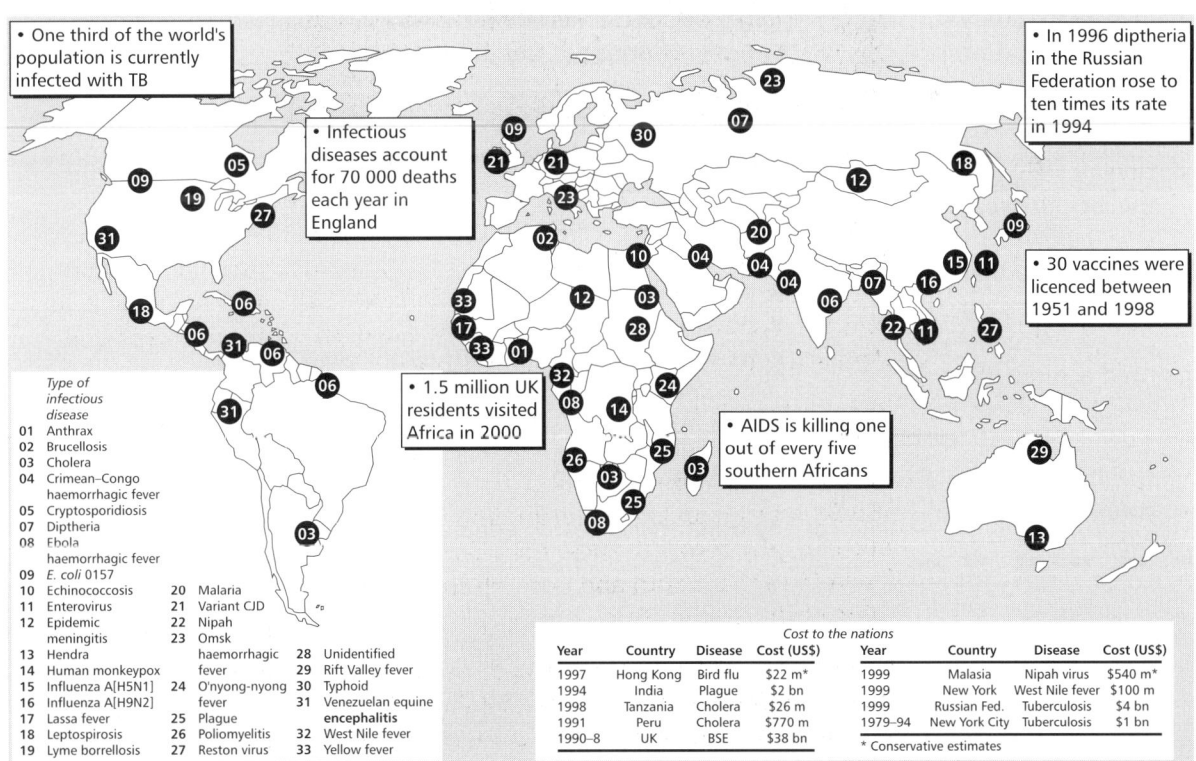

Figure 2.7 Outbreaks of infectious disease around the world (1994–2001)

THE WORLD OF DISEASE   27

Whilst the record of smallpox is a heartening one, there remain other infectious diseases which, whilst they may have been largely eradicated from MEDCs, persist as serious killers in LEDCs. Typhoid and cholera are two such diseases. The hope is that the steps already taken against those diseases in the North can be replicated in the South – the sooner the better. However, should we require any reminder of the need to be ever vigilant about infectious disease, then a look at **2.7** should do the trick. It draws our attention to some of the 30 new and nasty diseases that have only been discovered in the past 30 years, plus some old 'favourites'.

This chapter has put the spotlight on diseases, both chronic and infectious. The global North–South divide can be seen in the overall pattern of disease. In the North, degenerative diseases are dominant, reinforced by exogenic circumstances such as lifestyles. In the South, infectious diseases dominate, with strong links to environmental conditions, particularly those partly created by human activities. The diseases considered have all been essentially physical ones. No attention has been paid to mental illnesses, despite the suffering that they cause worldwide – and nowhere more so than in the North. They have been omitted from the discussion because they are rarely fatal. But that is not to suggest that mental illness does not have a strong bearing on welfare and well-being.

Review

7 How might you explain the fact that infectious diseases are the main killers in LEDCs?

8 Explain how each of the bulleted factors in the case study is contributing to the spread of dengue fever.

9 Do you think that the victory over smallpox was a 'one-off', or that the same strategy can be successfully used against other infectious diseases, such as cholera and typhoid? Justify your viewpoint.

Enquiry

1 Investigate how the urban and rural areas of the UK differ in terms of disease. Refer to **2.2** and **2.4** as a starting-point. Suggest reasons for the differences.

2 Research one of the following diseases shown in **2.7**: Ebola (08), *E. coli* 0157 (09), lassa fever (17) and Lyme's disease (19). Pay particular attention to:

- where it occurs
- possible causal links
- how it is transmitted
- its seriousness, in terms of disability or death.

You might start a web search at:

http://www.google.com

or any other major search engine.

CHAPTER 3

The spread of disease

Diseases are highly geographical in that they all have spatial distributions. Their incidence varies from place to place. The first stage in much medical research is to identify that spatial distribution, but at the same time to take into account frequency (**morbidity**). Having dealt with the 'where' and 'to what extent', the investigation will most likely move on to try to discover factors that seem to have influenced the distribution pattern and frequency. Researchers might then compare the current pattern and frequency with earlier ones, in order to establish whether or not there have been significant changes. Much interest will now focus on the process of spatial diffusion. Answers will have to be sought to key questions such as:

- In which directions has the disease spread?
- To what extent?
- At what speed?
- And how?

The first case study has been included as a warning, at the outset, that the explanation of morbidity is rarely very straightforward. It shows how difficult it can be to establish what, at first sight, might seem a fairly obvious causal link. Even with the help of the latest medical science and technology, experts still cannot agree on an explanation. Perhaps this is yet another case of multiple causality!

Case study: Seeking Sellafield's deadly secret

It was back in 1983 when the media first drew attention to an unusually large number of cases of childhood leukaemia near the Sellafield nuclear reprocessing plant in West Cumbria. All the children suffering from the disease were born in the nearby village of Seascale. Was the nuclear plant to blame? If so, what were the causal links?

- Some scientists were convinced that the high incidence of leukaemia was a direct result of contamination on nearby beaches. For them, it was the radioactivity of Sellafield's outfall into the Irish Sea that was to blame.
- Others argued that the exposure to radioactivity occurred because of the consumption of local seafood and locally produced foodstuffs.
- Still others thought that the causal link was the high radiation doses that the fathers of those children received in their work at the Sellafield plant.

> **Review**
>
> 1 Check that you have not forgotten the meaning of **morbidity**.
>
> 2 Which of the Sellafield explanations impresses you most? Do you think that the concept of **multiple causality** has something to offer here?

- At one time, it was thought by some that babies had contracted the disease as a result of crawling on floors that were coated with radioactive dust.
- Most recently, a number of scientists have suggested that there is no link at all with the reprocessing plant. Their argument is based on the idea that the leukemia may be caused by a viral infection rather than exposure to radioactivity. It has been noted elsewhere in areas of substantial in-migration (as was the case with Sellafield in the late 1950s and early 1960s) that in-migrants often bring 'new' viruses with them. If the local population has had no previous exposure to the introduced viruses, then they are likely to have little or no immunity. In short, the impact of any imported virus can be quite considerable. We might refer to this as the **population mixing** hypothesis (bear it in mind when you read the case study on page 37).

SECTION A

The role of the natural environment

When trying to explain the incidence of a disease, an obvious starting-point is to establish whether or not there are any links with the natural environment. When doing this, it is important to bear in mind the concept introduced in Chapter 2, namely that of **multiple causality**. In other words, the situation may well not be one of a simple cause-and-effect nature. Let us first take a look at **3.1**, prepared by the World Health Organization (WHO), which indicates potential relationships between various environmental exposure situations and the prevalence of particular health conditions.

Water

The two aspects of the physical environment that most immediately affect people are the quality of water and air (**3.1**). It is widely recognised that there are many different infectious diseases related to water in a variety of ways. Such diseases can be grouped into four categories:

- **Faecal–oral diseases** – these are spread by highly contagious micro-organisms. This category includes cholera and typhoid. Whilst it is true that they are transmitted through drinking water, all of the infections in this group can also be passed on by contaminated food, fingers, utensils and even clothes.
- **Water-washed skin and eye diseases** – these have little to do with water quality, but tend to prevail where water is in short supply. Some of the diseases in this group can have very serious effects; for example, trachoma can end in blindness.
- **Water-based diseases** – these are caused by parasitic worms that cannot pass directly from one person to another, but must first develop in another animal that lives in water, usually a snail. The most famous

Health conditions	Exposure situations					
	Polluted air	Excreta and household wastes	Polluted water or deficiencies in water management	Polluted food	Unhealthy housing	Global environmental change
Acute respiratory infections	●				●	
Diarrhoeal diseases		●	●	●		
Malaria and other vector-borne diseases		●	●	●		●
Other infections		●	●	●	●	
Cancer	●			●		●
Cardiovascular disorders	●					●
Mental disorders					●	
Chronic respiratory diseases	●					●
Injuries and poisonings	●		●	●	●	●

Figure 3.1 Potential relationships between exposure situations and health conditions

of these diseases is bilharzia, which is caught by wading or swimming in infected water.

- **Water-related insect-vector diseases** – these are spread by insects that breed in water (such as mosquitos) or bite near to rivers. The different types of insect responsible for each disease prefer different bodies of water in which to breed. One type, for example, breeds in the water tanks on large buildings in Indian cities and transmits a particular form of malaria. Another likes septic tanks and puddles of waste water, and transmits a disfiguring condition known as elephantiasis.

The catalogue of water-borne diseases clearly suggests that a proper water supply is vital to good health. The message of **3.2** is that there are many LEDCs in which large sections of the population are deprived of safe water and adequate sanitation. Of course, there will areas within those countries where the situation is even worse than indicated by the national means.

THE SPREAD OF DISEASE

Figure 3.2 Access to safe water and adequate sanitation in selected countries (1996)

Country	% of population with access to safe water	% of population with access to adequate sanitation
Afghanistan	12	8
Cambodia	36	14
Central African Republic	38	27
Ethiopia	25	19
Gambia	48	37
Haiti	37	25
Madagascar	34	41
Malawi	37	6
Papua New Guinea	28	22
Somalia	31	43
Sudan	50	22
Zambia	27	64

Case study: The malaria monster

Malaria is an infectious disease caused by the presence of protozoa (known as *Plasmodia*) in the red blood cells. It is a vector-borne disease transmitted by the blood-sucking, female *Anopheles* mosquito. It is confined to tropical and subtropical regions, particularly to ill-drained areas.

When the mosquito bites, malarial parasites picked up from the last human victim carrying the disease are injected into the blood stream and migrate to the liver and other organs, where they multiply. After incubating for up to 10 months, the parasites return to the blood stream and invade the red blood cells. Rapid multiplication of the parasites ruptures the cells, causing fever, shivering and sweating. When the next batch of parasites is released, the symptoms reappear. The intervals between bouts of fever vary with different types of malaria – four main types are recognised. Severe forms of malaria cause both liver and kidney failure, as well as brain and lung complications.

There are between 300 and 500 million new cases of malaria reported annually, 90 per cent of them in Africa. About 270 million people are believed to be infected at any one time. Up to 2 million people die every year from malaria and its complications, and over 2.4 billion people, almost half the world's population, are at risk of contracting the disease.

The battle against malaria has proceeded on two fronts:

- By treatment of the habitat where the *Anopheles* mosquito breeds (remember that there are many species of mosquito, but it is only this

Figure 3.3 Spraying the mosquito with DDT

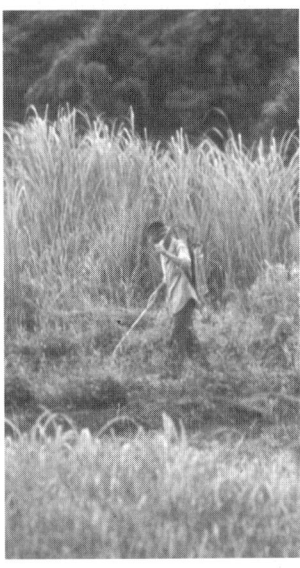

one that carries the disease, and then only the females). This has involved either draining the offending swampy areas or spraying them intensively with DDT and similar chemicals (**3.3**).

- By encouraging those at risk to take preventive medication. This usually involves either a daily dose of chloroquin or a weekly dose of paludrin – sometimes both. Unless treated in its initial stage, there is no cure for malaria. Once fully contracted, malaria is in the body for life.

The fact is that, for all the action programmes, malaria remains one of the most prevalent and devastating parasitic diseases to afflict the human race. Major setbacks have been encountered in the fight against the disease:

- The resistance of the mosquito to DDT and other chemicals continues to grow.
- There is also a growing resistance to the drugs taken by people to prevent them catching it. This applies particularly to the strain known as *Plasmodia falciparum*, which affects the brain. At present, only mefloquine is capable of providing adequate protection, but this drug has received bad publicity as a result of the side-effects suffered by some people. Unwisely, by choosing not to take this medicine, people run the risk of contracting a particularly lethal strain of malaria.
- The cost of anti-malaria drugs is clearly a problem in LEDCs, and a serious obstacle to ever achieving the ultimate end-game in the battle – namely, a population in which not a single person is carrying the disease. It only needs one carrier and one female *Anopheles* mosquito, and the vicious circle that spreads the disease is set in motion again.
- Adding to the tale of woe is the recent discovery that global warming is encouraging malaria to creep up into mountain areas in countries such as Kenya, Ethiopia and Papua New Guinea. Mosquitoes are now transmitting the disease above 2000 m where, previously, people have not been taking precautions against malaria.

Malaria is one of the most intriguing of the so-called water-borne diseases. It is one of the South's biggest killers. Having read the above case study, what do you think is the precise nature of malaria's relationship with water? Is the link simply that waterlogged conditions favour the disease, or is it that those conditions favour the vector mosquito? Or does the answer lie in both? The truth of the matter is that scientists are still uncertain as to how the malaria parasites developed in the first instance. It is even possible that they did not evolve in watery areas.

Air

What should also be becoming apparent is the possibility that some diseases are related to the human impact on the natural environment rather than to the natural environment itself. The pollution of water clearly has much to answer for, particularly with regard to the first of the four categories of water-borne disease (faecal–oral; **3.1**). Similarly, the pollution of air has particularly adverse consequences for human health There are well established links between air quality and the incidence of respiratory diseases, perhaps most notably bronchitis. It is in cities that air pollution reaches its highest levels, because of the concentrated burning of fossil fuels and the agglomeration of manufacturing (**3.4**). Air pollution is something that is suffered by rich and poor alike.

City	Population (m)	Total suspended particulates	Sulphur dioxide	Nitrogen dioxide
		(microgrammes per cumec)		
Bucharest (Romania)	2.1	82	10	71
Guayaquil (Ecuador)	2.3	127	15	n.d.
Munich (Germany)	2.3	48	8	53
Nagpur (India)	2.1	185	6	13
Vancouver (Canada)	2.0	29	14	37
Zhengzhou (China)	2.1	474	63	95

Figure 3.4 Air pollution in selected cities with populations around 2 million (1996)

Case study: Cooking smoke a silent killer

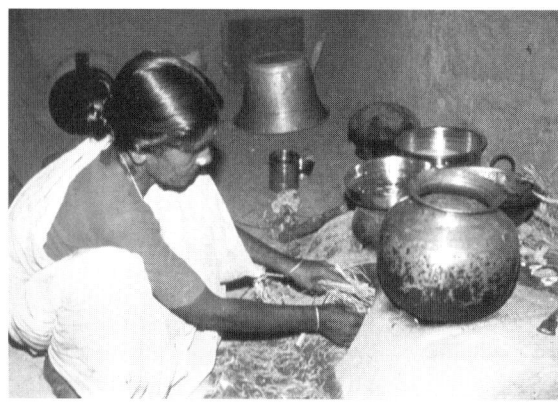

Figure 3.5 Cooking by open fire in an LEDC

Billions of dollars have been spent on research into the harmful effects of outdoor air pollution. Comparatively little has been done to protect human health from indoor air pollution, other than that resulting from smoking tobacco. Wood, stubble, dung and grass are used daily in about half of the world's households as energy for cooking and heating. In most parts of the South, they are burnt in open fires or inefficient stoves, in poorly ventilated kitchens (**3.5**). The result is a toll in ill health and death that is far greater than that associated with outdoor air pollution.

Smoke from burning biomass contains many harmful constituents, including particulates and carbon monoxide. Exposure to these substances can cause serious respiratory infections, as well as pneumonia, tuberculosis and cataracts. Coal smoke especially contains sulphur and nitrogen oxides and hydrocarbons that can lead to cancer.

The WHO estimates that about 2500 million people in the world, particularly women and children, are exposed to excessive levels of indoor air pollution. Most of this pollution comes from burning biomass and coal indoors in ovens that are badly designed and lack proper chimneys. African countries and India have the worst record for indoor pollution in rural homes, while the record for urban homes is worst in Latin America, India and China.

Clearly, pollution is one form of environmental abuse that has a range of consequences for disease. The next case study illustrates another – 'unnatural' exposure to an element of the natural environment.

Case study: Malignant melanoma

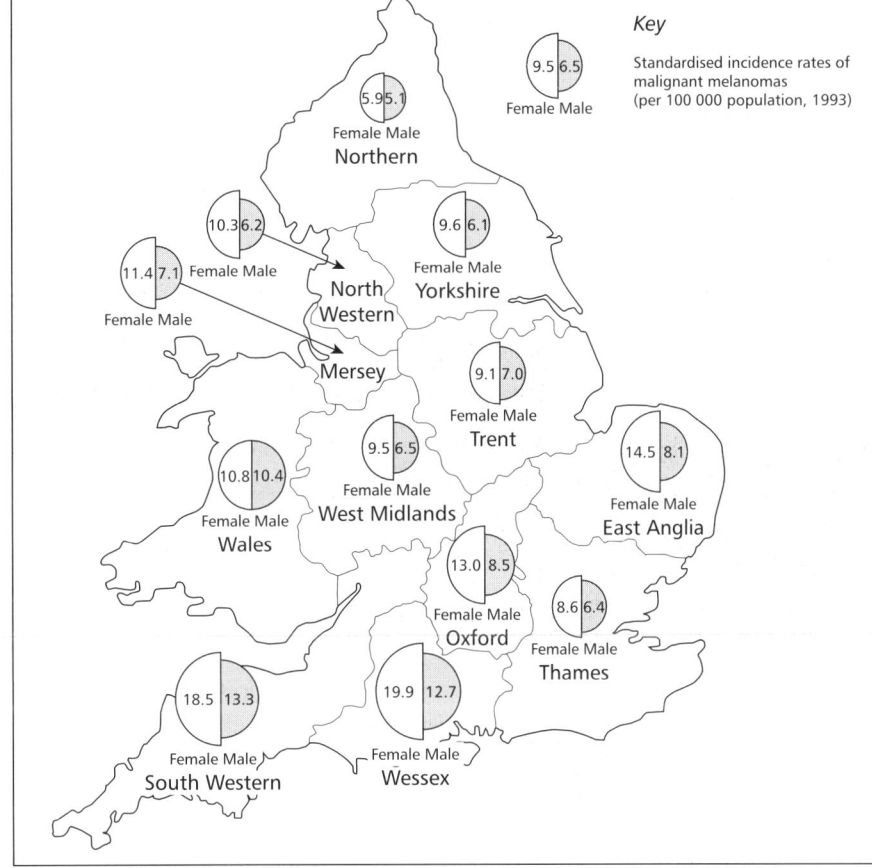

Figure 3.6 Standardised incidence rates for malignant melanoma in England and Wales, by health authorities

This is a form of skin cancer that is thought to be related to ultraviolet radiation. The number of cases rose significantly during the second half of the 20th century (**3.6**). Research suggests that, unlike other forms of skin cancer, the risk factor is not regular outdoor exposure to sunlight. The cause appears to lie in the intermittent but intense exposure of unacclimatised skin to sunlight. Increased incidence and mortality are thought to be due to behavioural changes, particularly the rise in overseas holidays taken by Britons and other Europeans in hotter climates. Also contributing is the current fashion for a sun-tanned appearance. Sun-block creams may well help to reduce the sunbather's risk of developing malignant melanomas, but they certainly do not remove it altogether.

Review

3 Explain some of the potential relationships shown in **3.1**.

4 Explain why it may be wrong to think of malaria as an environmental disease.

5 To what extent do you agree with the view that reducing water pollution is a simple way of reducing the spread of disease?

6 Write a brief analytical account based on **3.6**.

SECTION B

The human hand

The picture that is beginning to emerge is as follows. Many of the infectious diseases that we might first think of as having 'natural' causes are in fact more attributable to people themselves. Misuse of the environment is one aspect of this; another is the creation of 'artificial' environments. The latter point is well made if we pause to consider the unhealthy nature of most human settlements, particularly the large urban ones (**3.4**). But even rural environments can become contaminated by disease.

In the cities of the South, it is common for one child in three to die before the age of five, and for virtually all infants, children and adults who survive to have disease burdens many times higher than they should have to carry. Diarrhoea, tuberculosis and respiratory infections (three of the global big killers) are generally much increased by overcrowding. Many accidental injuries happen when there are three or more persons living in each small room in shelters made from flammable materials, and there is little chance of providing occupants with protection from open fires or stoves. Hence the problem in so many LEDC cities is not the high densities but, rather, the poor quality of the housing, and the failure to provide treated piped water and safe waste disposal.

Case study: Killing pests and people

Evidence indicates that millions of farm workers, rural households and consumers are still exposed to dangerous levels of pesticides. It is not only farm workers who are affected as they apply something like 100 000 tonnes of dangerous organo-chlorine pesticides, mainly in the LEDCs. The use of such chemicals is now banned in many MEDCs, but the ban has not stopped manufacturers in those countries from marketing their pesticides to the Third World. Up to 30 per cent of farmers in Latin America show damage to their neuro-muscular system as a result of pesticide poisoning. Only 10–15 per cent of pesticides reach their targets on the farm. The rest is dispersed through the air, soil and water, some of it only over many years. Remember too that pesticides are used intensively in the fight against malaria and dengue fever (**3.3**). So here is a situation in which one disease is being conquered, but others encouraged.

Some of this straying pesticide gets into dairy products. For example, in parts of Mexico and Argentina, most butter and cheese contains pesticide residues. Research among Inuit people in Canada found that the consumption of pesticide-contaminated fish and marine mammals were affecting breast milk. This in turn was depressing the immune system in babies, thus exposing them to infections such as meningitis. Similar impacts on the immune systems of farmers and people living in rural areas have left them more at risk in terms of developing cancer.

The second case study in this section serves to underline the unhealthy nature of the most human of all environments, towns and cities. It also provides a link to the next section, which focuses on the role of people in spreading disease.

Case study: The unhealthy Tropics?

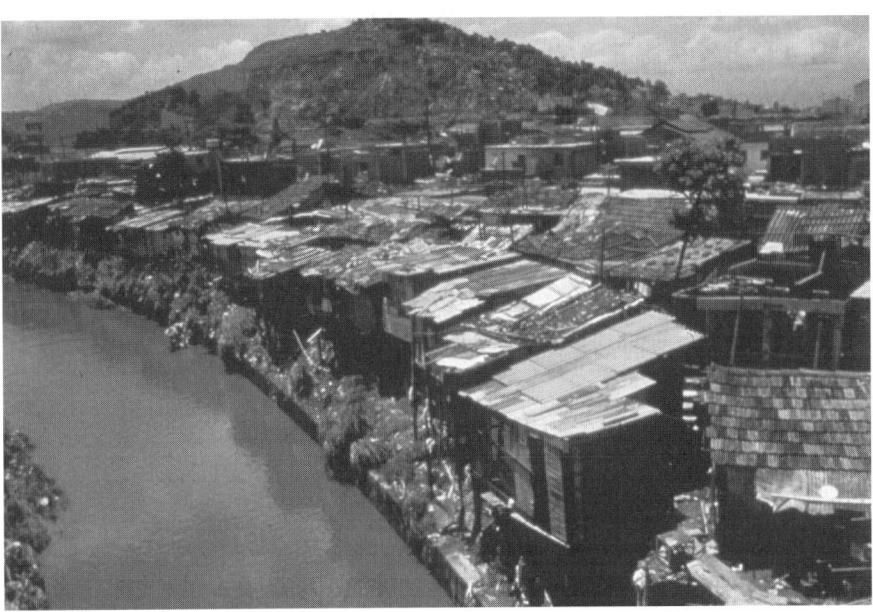

Figure 3.7 Shanty housing in the Tropics; an ideal breeding ground for Europe's disease exports

The Tropics are frequently perceived today as an inherently unhealthy place. Despite the catalogue of diseases presented in **2.6** (pages 24–25), it would be wrong to think that tropical areas are rife with killer diseases. More than that, there is evidence that these areas were healthier before their colonisation by Europeans. Early travellers in Africa, for example, commented favourably on the physical well-being of the native peoples. It was Europe that was essentially disease-ridden and it was the Europeans who took the diseases abroad, as for example to the Americas. Here, the Amerindian population died in their millions because they had no immunity to the introduced pathogens. The diseases now found in the Tropics, such as TB, cholera, leprosy and bubonic plague, were – until relatively recently – widespread in urban Europe. Those diseases disappeared in Europe because of improved living conditions and nutrition. Having been 'exported' to the Tropics, the same diseases persist today, mostly noticeably in towns and cities where – as in Europe 200 years ago – high population densities and pollution create an environment in which infectious diseases flourish and spread with amazing speed (**3.7**).

Review

7 Is it high densities that create the health problems of cities?

8 Pesticides – good or bad? Produce a two-column list of the arguments.

9 What hypothesis about the spread of disease may be supported by the case study of the Tropics?

SECTION C

Modes of transmission

In the case of infectious diseases in particular, distributions can change quite significantly, expanding and intensifying during **epidemics** (sudden outbreaks marked by rapid spreading). The distributions of non-infectious diseases also change, but usually much more slowly.

Six basic organisms are involved in infectious diseases. These are shown in **3.8** along with the five main modes of disease transmission. The case studies of typhoid and dengue fever in the previous chapter have already illustrated two different modes of transmission. With the former, the bacteria are spread through the contamination of food and water. With the latter, a particular species of mosquito is the culprit. Because of this, dengue fever – and malaria too – are referred to as **vector-borne diseases**.

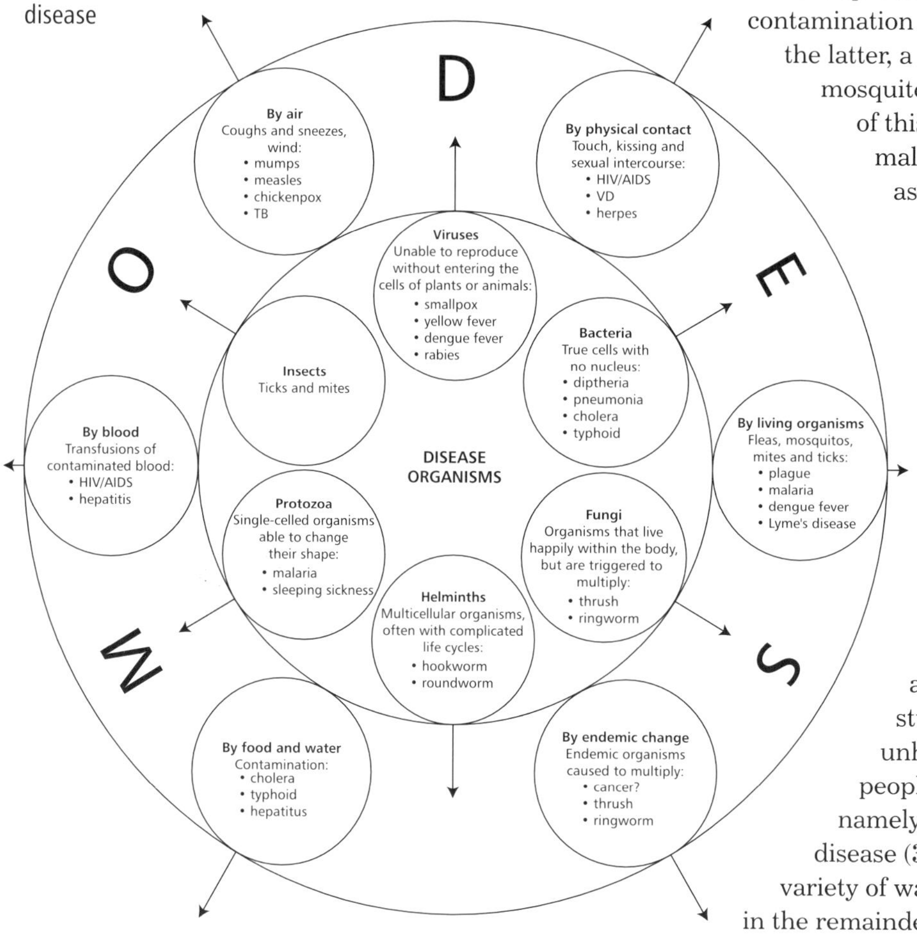

Figure 3.8 The transmission of disease

Diagram showing DISEASE ORGANISMS at centre, with MODES arranged around:

- **By air** – Coughs and sneezes, wind: mumps, measles, chickenpox, TB
- **By physical contact** – Touch, kissing and sexual intercourse: HIV/AIDS, VD, herpes
- **By living organisms** – Fleas, mosquitos, mites and ticks: plague, malaria, dengue fever, Lyme's disease
- **By endemic change** – Endemic organisms caused to multiply: cancer?, thrush, ringworm
- **By food and water** – Contamination: cholera, typhoid, hepatitus
- **By blood** – Transfusions of contaminated blood: HIV/AIDS, hepatitis

Disease organisms:
- **Viruses** – Unable to reproduce without entering the cells of plants or animals: smallpox, yellow fever, dengue fever, rabies
- **Bacteria** – True cells with no nucleus: diptheria, pneumonia, cholera, typhoid
- **Fungi** – Organisms that live happily within the body, but are triggered to multiply: thrush, ringworm
- **Helminths** – Multicellular organisms, often with complicated life cycles: hookworm, roundworm
- **Protozoa** – Single-celled organisms able to change their shape: malaria, sleeping sickness
- **Insects** – Ticks and mites

The human role in disease is not just one of victim. We have already established another in the sense that people can inadvertently create the conditions that nurture certain diseases. This might be by pollution, by behaving irresponsibly (remember the malignant melanoma and the pesticides case studies) or by building unhealthy settlements. But people play a third role; namely, as transmitters of disease (**3.8**). This they do in a variety of ways that will be illustrated in the remainder of this chapter.

Case study: Travel, terrorism and the transmission of disease

The UK's Chief Medical Officer has recently warned that long-haul travel and international terrorism have put the country in the front line of dozens of new and incurable diseases. The danger is now thought to be so great that the British government is setting up a new agency to counteract the threat.

The vogue for long-haul travel and holidays in distant exotic locations is greatly increasing the risks of Britons catching deadly infections. In 2001, 1.5 million British residents visited Africa and nearly 2 million went to Asia. Six million Britons travelled to malarial areas; 2000 of them returned from holiday with the disease. Incredibly, it is estimated that one in five of such travellers do not take any anti-malarial precautions. One million people a week cross a border between an MEDC and an LEDC. But it is not just a matter of British travellers returning home infected. Diseases such as typhoid (see page 25) are being brought into the country by overseas visitors.

The move to set up the agency was also prompted by the terrorist attacks of 11 September 2001, and the subsequent threat of biological, chemical and even nuclear attacks by Islamic extremists.

Review

10 Check that you understand the difference between a **viral** and a **bacterial** infection.

11 Which of the five modes of disease transmission shown in **3.8** do you think is the most significant? Give your reasons.

12 'If there were no people, there would be no disease.' Discuss.

SECTION D

The HIV/AIDS pandemic

Having introduced the idea of people as transmitters of disease, perhaps it is time to start discussing one of today's 'big killers' – HIV/AIDS. Acquired immune-deficiency syndrome (AIDS) is an incurable disease that was first identified in 1980. It results from infection by the human immuno-deficiency virus (HIV). By gradually destroying the body's defences against disease, the way is opened up for a whole range of opportunistic infections to occur. Therefore, 'AIDS' is something of an umbrella term to cover all of those infections, one or more of which will ultimately be the cause of death. It could be pneumonia, malaria, typhoid or whatever.

Although HIV is highly infectious, it has a long incubation period, of at least six years. It is essentially a sexually transmitted disease, but it can be passed on in other ways: through contaminated blood or blood products, contaminated hypodermic needles, and even from mother to child during childbirth.

Figure **3.9** gives a snapshot of the global distribution of HIV/AIDS in 1997. Since then, the pattern has not changed a great deal, except for an alarming spread into and across Russia. What has altered are the prevalence figures and the number of deaths annually. In 2001 alone, the death toll was estimated as 3 million. The figure is staggering and is expected to continue to rise. The scale is such that researchers now refer to the AIDS **pandemic** (a massive, worldwide outbreak). At the end of 2001, an estimated 40 million people globally were living with HIV. Since the pandemic began, more than 60 million people have been infected by the virus. HIV/AIDS is now the leading cause of death in sub-Saharan Africa. Worldwide, it is now the fourth biggest killer.

The two case studies of AIDS that follow illustrate how HIV is spread by different types of physical contact. But both clearly underline the importance of migration, transport and lifestyles as agents that foster the spectacular spread of this and other killer viruses.

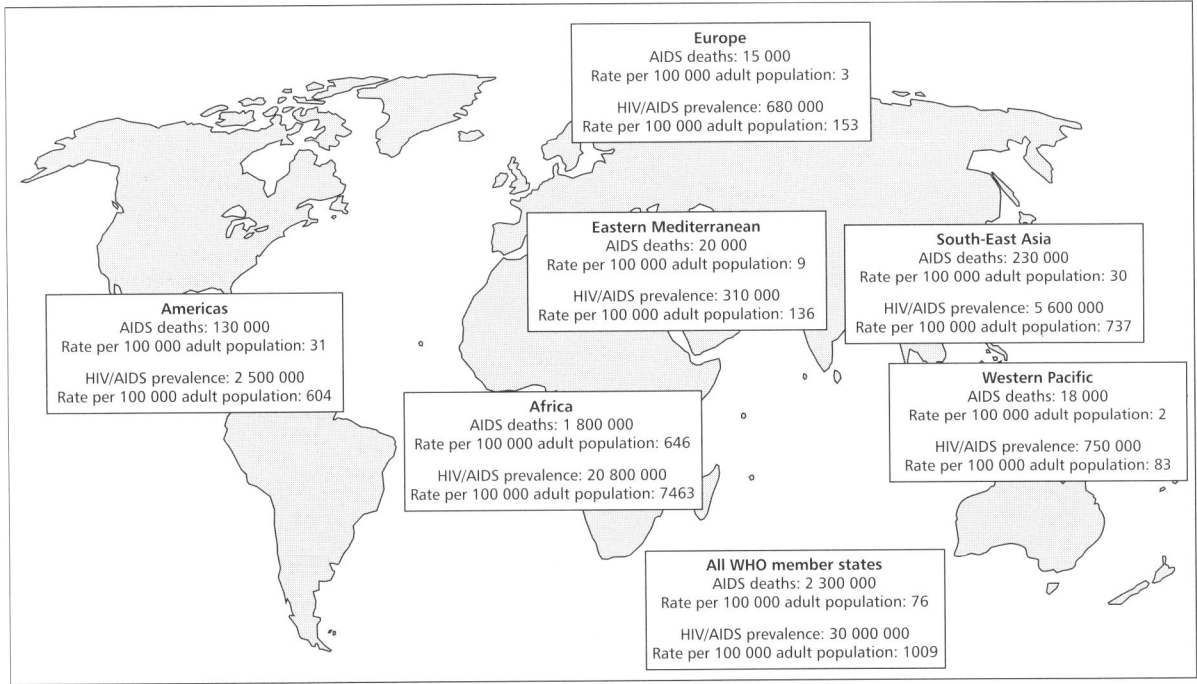

Figure 3.9 AIDS deaths and HIV/AIDS prevalence among adults aged 15–49 by global region (1997)

Case study: AIDS on the march in Uganda

The occurrence of AIDS in Uganda provides a simple illustration of what is involved in a geographical investigation of disease. The first step is to collect data that are as reliable as possible about the incidence of the disease and to map the distribution pattern (**3.10**). The next step is to attempt to explain that pattern by means of hypothesis-testing and regression analysis.

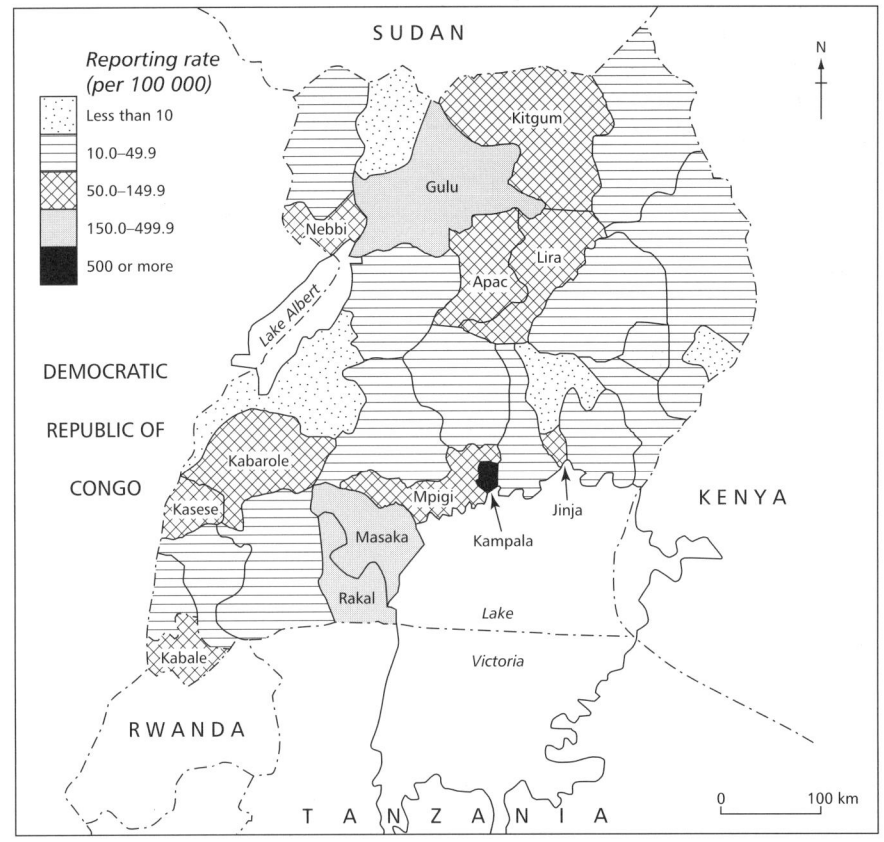

Figure 3.10 The incidence of AIDS in Uganda

The search for an explanation of the spatial pattern in **3.10** was based on the established fact that HIV leading to the onset of AIDS is spread by sexual intercourse (particularly with prostitutes) and the sharing of drug needles. In the case of Uganda, three hypotheses were tested:

- That areas of high in- and out-migration have higher AIDS rates. This is based on the idea that the AIDS virus 'trickles down' from urban to rural areas via workers returning home to rural areas from their urban workplaces. Similarly, those areas (largely urban) that are demanding labour may also be expected to show high rates.
- That high rates of AIDS occur along the roads used by those migrants who are moving between rural and urban areas.
- That the Ugandan military has played a significant role in the spread of the disease. There is evidence from other African countries of high rates of HIV infection amongst existing and former soldiers.

The regression coefficients (R^2) were calculated as 5.7 per cent, 17.4 per cent and 43.0 per cent, respectively.

Thus only the third hypothesis contributed much to a possible explanation of the spatial variation in AIDS rates. With only two-thirds of the variation explained by the three hypothesis, clearly the search for other contributory actors continues (see the China case study below). But what has been demonstrated here is a research methodology of 'describe and explain' to discover possible causal links.

THE SPREAD OF DISEASE

Case study: AIDS in China – the 'Road of Death'

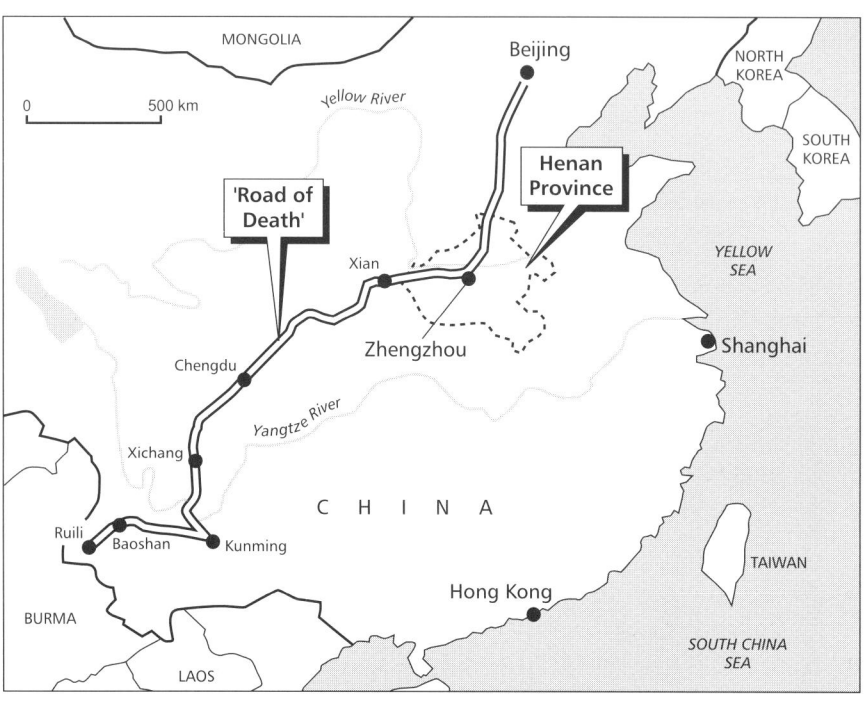

Figure 3.11 The 'Road of Death', China

China, by far the most populous country in the world, is facing an AIDS epidemic that has already led to the infection of 80 per cent of the population in some areas. In fact, in places, particularly in Henan Province, infection rates are higher than any in Africa.

The spread of the disease has been particularly rampant along a main road that runs across virtually the whole of the country in a south-west–north-east direction (**3.11**). What is now known as the 'Road of Death' starts in the heroin fields on the border with Burma and ends in Beijing. The Chinese drug trade is booming and has been doing so for many years. All along the 1500 mile (2400 km) route, there are thousands of dealers and hundreds of thousands of addicts, most of whom are taking heroin intravenously. The sharing of needles has helped a phenomenal transmission of HIV.

But other factors have played their part. Each year, millions of migrant workers (the 'foot soldiers' of China's economic miracle) pass along this route. Being away from home for months or years, many sleep with prostitutes in worker camps and sell drugs to supplement meagre wages. Another contributor to the nightmare scenario has been the custom that developed when China took its first step towards a market economy. Having been deprived of state subsidies, and in order to support their families, poor farmers began to sell blood to blood banks. Without proper screening of donors, HIV-contaminated blood was allowed to 'pollute' great pools of blood assembled for the extraction of the plasma used in pharmaceuticals. Just think of the consequences of such carelessness! Finally, the whole situation has been made worse by the fact that, up until the middle of 2001, the Chinese government had always denied the existence of AIDS in the country. Certainly, nothing had been done before then to warn the people or to provide any guidance about avoiding the disease.

What will be the outcome of this dreadful convergence of circumstances?

The general tone of these two case studies is inescapably depressing. Adding to this is the fact that AIDS is not only decimating the population of much of Africa, where whole families have been wiped out, millions of children orphaned and relatively few fit people left to work. AIDS is also threatening to become a major killer in the North. Russia is already well down that road. Can modern medicine do more for sufferers in this part of the world? Is there a cure in sight? Will research ever come up with a preventive drug that would allow a global mass vaccination programme? Clearly, the longer it takes to put in place effective preventive measures (be it discovering drugs or changing lifestyles), the more millions will be added to the list of victims! One can only speculate about the likely long-term impact of this AIDS pandemic. Will it create a huge population implosion?

Finally, as a postscript, it should be noted that chronic or non-infectious diseases also change their distributions. The changes are not brought about so much by transmission and diffusion but, rather, by processes such as a general ageing of a population, a shift in lifestyles or some small change in the environment.

Three broad conclusions are to be drawn from the ground covered in this chapter:

- There are relatively few diseases that are directly linked to specific natural environments. If they do occur, links tend to be indirect, as with malaria and dengue fever and their all-important vector mosquitos.
- The spread of infectious diseases has been encouraged by human abuse of the natural environment. Just recall how many rivers, lakes and ponds are still treated no better than as sewers, cesspools and dumps. It is little wonder that water-borne diseases are so prevalent.
- Built environments, particularly towns and cities, can so easily become disease hot spots. Human settlements do seem to have developed their own portfolio of diseases, including illnesses in the home. But, as some of the case studies illustrate, the human hand in the spread of disease and death also reaches into rural areas and beyond national frontiers – be it by road, farm machinery, migrants, tourists, terrorists or casual personal contacts.

Review

13 Be sure that you remember the salient features of the global distribution shown in 3.9.

14 Write a brief account highlighting the essential features of the distribution pattern shown in 3.10.

15 Identify the various factors encouraging the spread of AIDS in China. To what extent is the situation different in Uganda?

16 Make a list of the ways in which people help to spread disease.

Enquiry

Using website sources, research one of the following diseases:

- tuberculosis
- cholera
- bilharzia.

Produce a report with the following headings:

- Global trends
- Distribution
- Contributory factors
- Checking the spread.

CHAPTER 4

The burden of disease

Disease can have a whole range of impacts – and not just on the victim. Particularly in epidemic and pandemic situations, the consequences can be both widespread and serious. They can be felt across the whole range of spatial scales, from the global to the local, and in the four main arenas identified in **4.1**; namely, the demographic, economic, social and environmental.

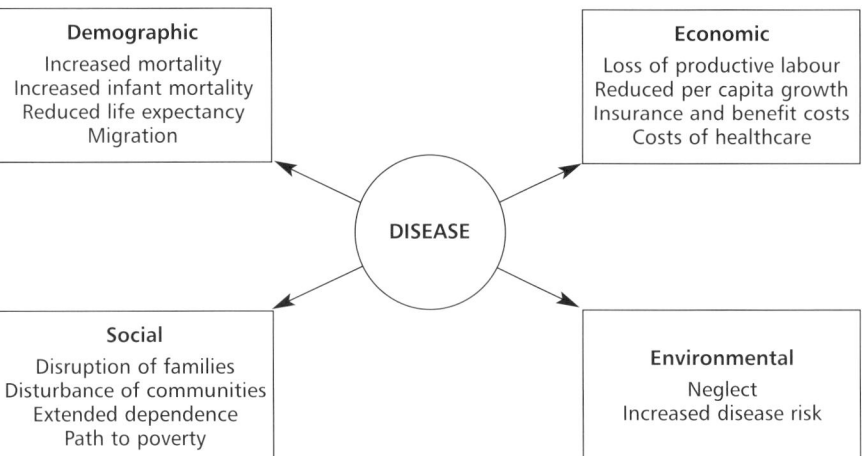

Figure 4.1 Some impacts of disease

SECTION A

Demographic impacts

Mortality and life expectancy

Of the four impact arenas, the demographic is the most obvious. A serious outbreak of disease is likely to boost the mortality rate, and if it persists for long enough, it might even have a lowering effect on life expectancy. That is the important difference between these two potential measures of the effects of disease on populations. Mortality rates provide a snapshot of a year's duration. A major epidemic of some fatal disease would certainly leave its mark on a year's death statistics. But remember that in any interpretation of mortality rates, it is necessary to take into account the overall age structure of the population (see standardised rates on page 8). In contrast, life expectancy provides a longer-term view of a population (annual perturbations are smoothed out) and age structure is automatically taken into account. What can be safely concluded from **4.2** or any more detailed map is that areas with below average life expectancy are those where persistent disease is cutting back the length of an average lifetime.

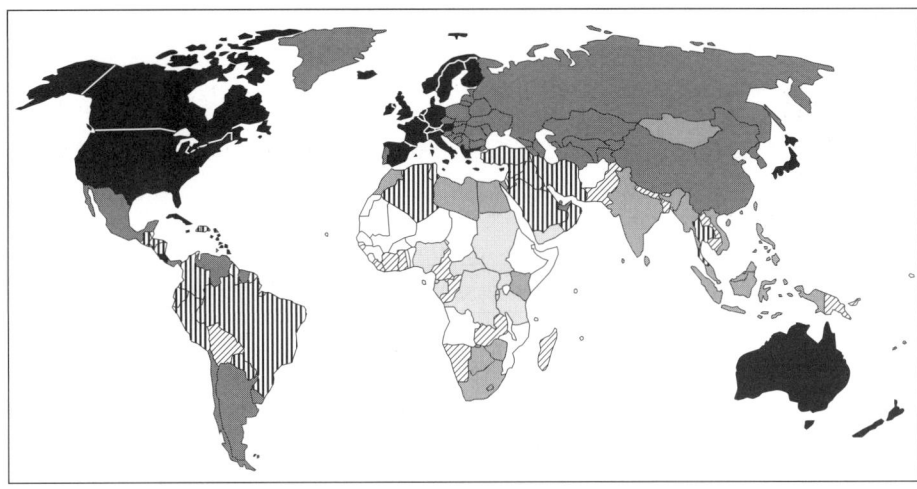

Figure 4.2 The global pattern of life expectancy (2000)

The message of **4.2** is all too clear: the populations of Africa and parts of South Asia are those suffering most from the burden of disease.

Age structure

Many diseases are age-specific in the sense that people within certain broad age ranges typically become their victims. Figure **4.3** tries to illustrate this important point in a highly generalised way. A few examples serve to push the point a little further.

Young children are probably the cohort that is most vulnerable to infectious disease. It takes time to acquire immunity, so that the first years of a life are particularly critical. Also helping to swell the **infant mortality rate** (the number of deaths of children aged under one year per 1000 live births) are genetic defects and injuries sustained during the birth process. The global infant mortality rate fell by over one-half during the second half of the 20th century. But at its present level of around 6 deaths per 1000 live births, it still means that some 8.5 million infants die each year before their first birthday. Infant mortality continues to chisel away at the base of the age pyramid (**4.3**). Despite the dramatic improvements, there remains a huge gap between the LEDCs and MEDCs (**4.4**). The infant mortality rate remains a respected measure of social affluence rather than just a reflection of the availability and quality of obstetric and antenatal care.

At present, HIV/AIDS hits the age pyramid

Figure 4.3 Age-related diseases

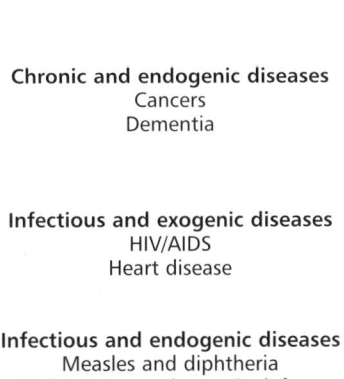

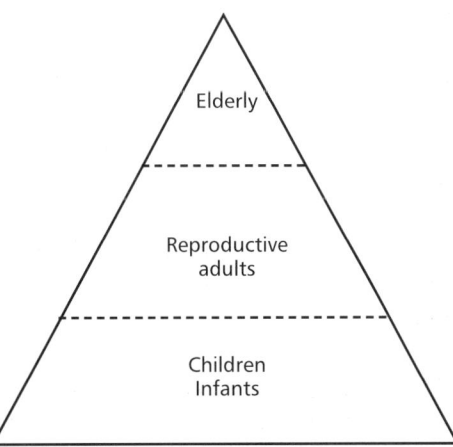

THE BURDEN OF DISEASE 45

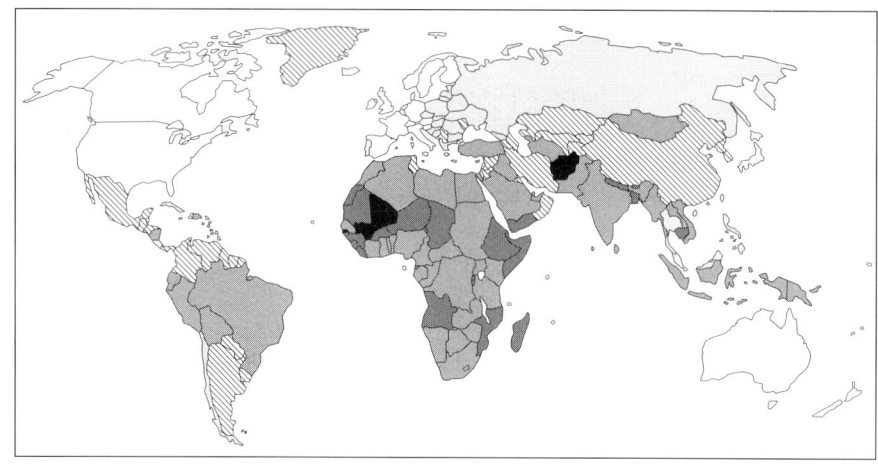

Figure 4.4 The global pattern of infant mortality (average 1990–1995)

higher up. It struck hardest at the young adult part of the population first, since the virus is transmitted most vigorously amongst the sexually active and drug users. More recently, the 'erosion' of the middle sections of the age pyramid has spread in two directions. It has moved up the pyramid, for the simple reason that many more people are not surviving into old age. It has also moved to the very base of the pyramid, for two separate reasons. First, more and more people are dying whilst still in their reproductive years. The result is a lowering of the birth rate. Secondly, there is the very sad fact that, before dying, AIDS victims often pass on the virus to their children. Only a small proportion of those HIV-positive children can expect to live much beyond the age of five. For this reason, the spread of AIDS is both undercutting the very base of the age pyramid and boosting rates of infant mortality that are already high, because of the general susceptibility of young children to a whole range of other diseases (**4.3**). In the Bahamas, it is estimated that 60 per cent of deaths among children under the age of five are due to AIDS, while in Zimbabwe the figure is 70 per cent.

What should be very clear by now is that the advent of AIDS has set in motion a chain of events, a vicious downward spiral, that has the potential to decimate whole populations (**4.5**). Not since the Black Death of the mid-14th century, which is estimated to have wiped out half of Europe's population, has a disease so threatened the world. It is beginning to look as though people have pressed the self-destruct button!

Figure 4.5 The vicious downward spiral in population created by AIDS

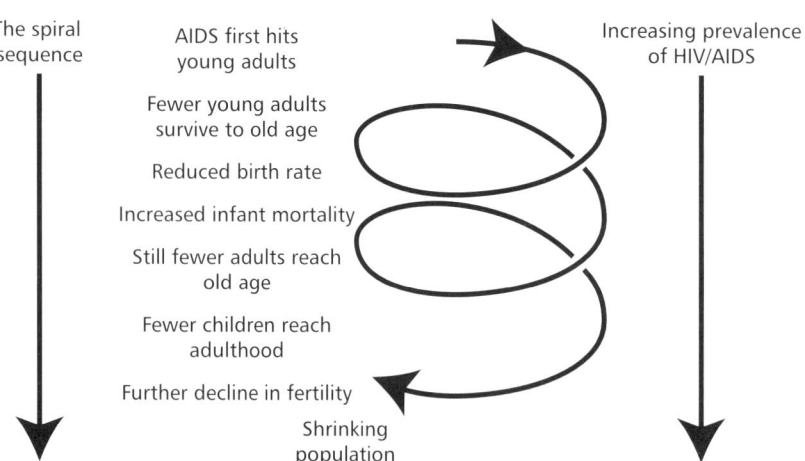

THE BURDEN OF DISEASE

Perhaps this is the point at which to introduce a more cheerful note in an otherwise wholly depressing discussion of the relationship between disease and people. It is simply that the waging of a successful battle against disease has resulted in the large elderly populations of many MEDCs, with their high levels of life expectancy. When elderly people eventually die, it is more likely that they have succumbed to chronic degenerative rather than to infectious diseases.

> **Review**
>
> 1 Why is life expectancy a better measure of the persistence of disease than the mortality rate?
>
> 2 What is meant by the term **age-related disease**?
>
> 3 Summarise the main features of the global pattern of infant mortality (**4.4**).
>
> 4 Check that you understand the links shown in **4.5**. Can you improve the diagram in any way?

SECTION B

Migration

There are a number of different links between disease and migration (**4.6**). With some of them, it is disease that impacts on migration. With others, the relationship works the other way round, with migration both spreading disease and increasing the risk of disease.

Disease as a push factor

First, and perhaps most obviously, disease can trigger migration (**4.6**). Way back in biblical times, it is possible that plagues were the push factor that prompted Moses to lead the Israelites out of Egypt. We can be more certain that in order to escape the Black Death, whole settlements infected by the disease were abandoned. There was a mass exodus to the countryside, where lower population densities meant a slowdown in the diffusion of the disease. Today, however, the situation is rather different. As a push factor, disease is well down the rankings – which are now probably topped by war and oppression.

A mode of transmission

The case studies of HIV/AIDS (pages 40 and 42) have clearly demonstrated the role played by the movement of people in the spread of the disease (**4.6**). Modern transport and the globalisation of tourism (short-term migration) are proving to be powerful diffusers of disease across international frontiers and from LEDCs to MEDCs. This was well

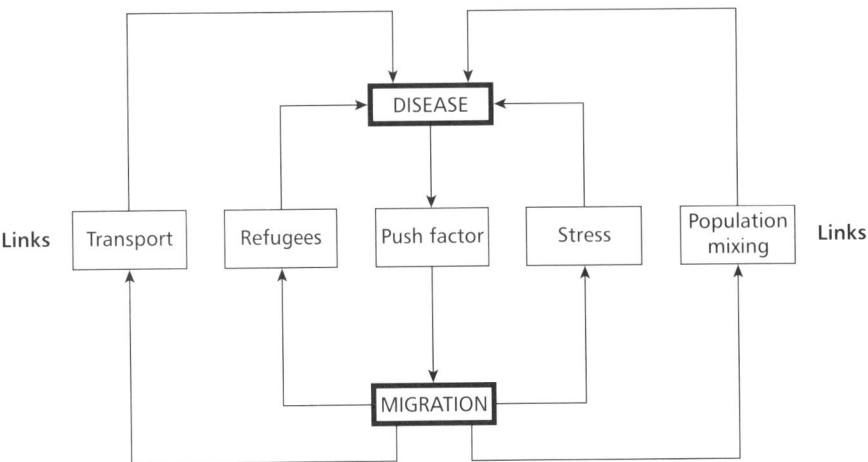

illustrated by the typhoid (page 25) and travel (page 38) case studies, and perhaps is also supported by that of Sellafield (page 29). It has also been shown (page 37) that a number of diseases that are now prevalent in LEDCs and in the New World were, in fact, carried there by European settlers.

Figure 4.6 The links between disease and migration

The health of the migrant

Consideration also needs to be given to the impact of migration on health (**4.6**). For example, there is evidence that migration, especially to a new country, leads to stress and depression. This arises from what is known as **alienation**, and the need to adjust to a new, and often very different, culture. Loneliness and homesickness are commonplace and can easily lead to alcohol and drug abuse, and even suicide. The data in **4.7** show that in Sweden the risk of suicide is significantly higher amongst women born outside the country than amongst women born in Sweden. In other words, migrants are more at risk.

Figure 4.7 The relative risk of suicide for Swedish-born and other women

Country of birth	Relative risk in Sweden	Relative risk in country of birth
Sweden	1.0	1.0
Finland	1.68	0.92
Poland	1.63	0.48
Russia	3.71	0.74
Germany	1.44	0.77
Hungary	3.39	1.84
Norway	0.99	0.57

It is the health of **refugees** (people who for various reasons are forced from their homes and seek refuge in another country) that frequently gives rise to concern. The dislocation can have drastic health consequences. Today's media all too often make us vividly aware of the impact of civil war, political persecution and ethnic cleansing on health, and indeed on life itself. Most recently, we have been shown the appalling conditions facing Afghan refugees.

Case study: The plight of Rwandan refugees

The population of Rwanda comprises two ethnic groups: the majority Hutus and the minority Tutsis. In July 1994 the Tutsis overturned the Hutu-dominated government. Fearing for their lives, over a million Hutus sought exile in neighbouring Zaire (now the Democratic Republic of Congo). In the following month nearly 50 000 refugees died, largely as a result of cholera and dysentery encouraged by the poor water supply and sanitation of the makeshift refugee camps. In addition, around 20 per cent of children aged under five were acutely malnourished. To make matters worse, the distribution of food and medical supplies was hindered by Rwandan military and political leaders.

Within a matter of months, nearly 3 million refugees had fled their homes, half of them moving across the borders to Zaire and Tanzania.

Review

5 How would you rate migration as a transmitter of disease compared with contaminated food and water?

6 Briefly explain the basic message contained in 4.7.

7 Is migration all bad news as far as disease is concerned?

Studies of refugee movements, particularly in Africa, have identified five main health impacts:

- The disruption of food production and healthcare. This leads to malnutrition. During the conflict in Somalia in 1992, nearly 75 per cent of the children under the age of five died from this cause.
- The overcrowding of refugee camps. Here, on top of food shortages, there are insanitary conditions. These lead to outbreaks of cholera, dysentery, hepatitis and measles.
- Increased sexual violence, particularly the rape of young girls and the exchange of sex for food. One obvious consequence here is the further spread of HIV.
- The trauma of watching people, often relatives and friends, being killed and mutilated.
- The sudden and chaotic mixing of people encourages the diffusion of new infections (back to the **population mixing** hypothesis mentioned in the Sellafield case study, page 29).

SECTION C

Wider consequences

Referring back to **4.1**, the repercussions of disease can be seen as reaching beyond demography to impact on the economy, society and the environment. The main aim of this section is simply to outline those consequences and to leave illustration to the following section, when once again the spotlight falls on HIV/AIDS.

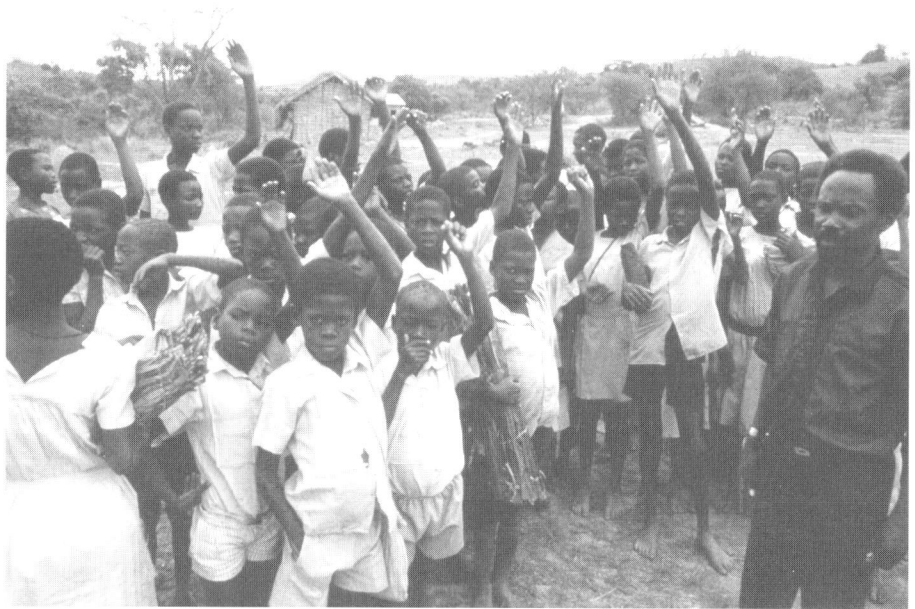

Figure 4.8 This picture was taken in the province of South Buganda, Uganda. The children here were asked to raise their hands if their parents had died from AIDS.

Review

8 Can you think of any more economic outcomes of disease?

9 Explain the link between disease and poverty.

10 Why should disease lead to neglect, and what diseases would you expect to be associated with neglect?

Economic

It is quite easy to think our way through a sequence of economic costs triggered by disease. If we make our starting-point the fact that people provide labour, the first and obvious consequence will be days of work lost through illness (**4.1**). Few employers can expect to run their businesses efficiently if the full labour requirement is not met. For most employees, absence from work means loss of income. Labour that is sick but remains at work because of a desperate need for money could well under-perform and do the firm few favours. Of course, some of the financial shortfall caused by illness can be met, as in a large number of MEDCs, by state sickness benefits or private insurance. But these are 'luxuries' that few LEDCs and few people in LEDCs can afford.

What we have traced so far is a sequence involving a single employee. Now think of an epidemic and scale up the consequences just outlined. At a regional and national level, the epidemic could well have a depressing effect on economic output (**4.1**). A reduction in per capita economic growth may well result. Meeting the costs incurred in tackling the disease and treating its victims will also put more strain on an already weakened economy.

Social

Disease can also have a whole range of social outcomes. Sickness and premature death all too frequently deprive families of either the wage-earner or much needed maternal care. Epidemics can clearly scale up the impact from the disruption of families to that of whole communities (**4.1**). In LEDCs, where care tends to be provided in the family rather than as an external service, the devastation caused by fatal diseases can result in a heavy burden of dependence for some. Families will be expected to look after distant relatives, whether they be orphaned children (**4.8**), a widow and her children or an elderly person who has lost all his or her children. Perhaps the worst of the social outcomes is that disease, with all its cost implications, can so easily push families down the slippery slope to poverty.

Environmental

Finally, we need to say a brief word about the environment. In studies of disease, the viewpoint is one of looking for causal links with some aspect of the environment. As we saw in **Chapter 3**, this is often to be found in some abuse or misuse of the environment. But does disease have an impact on the environment? The short answer is 'not a lot', except again possibly in epidemic situations, where neglect may be an outcome. This, in turn, can impact on the human environment. The neglect of farmland, of water supplies, of waste disposal and of dwellings could all lead to a worsening of the general health situation. Therefore the impact turns on itself in a self-perpetuating way.

SECTION D — Repercussions of the AIDS pandemic

Reference has already been made to the impact of AIDS on mortality rates and life expectancy (**4.5**). But the pandemic is having wider repercussions of the types outlined in the previous section. Those repercussions are being increasingly felt in many countries across the world. Southern Africa continues to be the worst affected area, with adult prevalence rates still rising in some areas. Here and elsewhere in countries already burdened by socio-economic problems, AIDS threatens human welfare, development progress and social stability on an unprecedented scale:

- It is estimated that per capita GDP in half the countries of sub-Saharan Africa is falling by between 0.5 and 1.2 per cent as a direct result of AIDS. By 2010, per capita GDP in some of the hardest hit countries may drop by 8 per cent and per capita consumption may fall even further. Calculations show that heavily infected countries could lose more than 20 per cent of GDP by 2020.
- Companies of all types face higher costs in training, insurance, benefits, absenteeism and illness. A survey of 15 firms in Ethiopia has shown that, over a five-year period, 53 per cent of all illnesses among staff were HIV-related.
- AIDS is setting in motion what are termed 'devastating cycles' of impoverishment. People at all income levels are vulnerable to the impact of HIV/AIDS, but the poor suffer most acutely. In Botswana, where adult HIV prevalence is over 35 per cent, one quarter of households can expect to lose an income-earner within the next 10 years. A rapid increase in the number of very poor and destitute families is anticipated. Per capita household income for the poorest quarter of households is expected to fall by 13 per cent. Every income-earner in this category can expect to take on four more dependants as a result of HIV/AIDS.
- According to a recent FAO Report, 7 million farm workers have died from AIDS-related causes since 1985, and 16 million more are expected to die in the next 20 years. Agricultural output – especially of staple foods – cannot be sustained. The prospect of food shortages and famine

is real. Some 20 per cent of rural families in Burkino Faso are estimated to have reduced their farming and even abandoned their farms altogether. Rural households in Thailand are already seeing their agricultural output shrink by half. In 15 per cent of these cases, children have been removed from school to take care of ill family members and to regain lost income. Here and elsewhere, it is girls who are withdrawn first.

- The number of African children who have lost their mother or both their parents to the pandemic numbered 12.1 million at the end of 2000 (**4.8**). The number of such orphans is forecast to more than double over the next decade.
- The pandemic is claiming large numbers of teachers, doctors, extension workers and other human resources. In some countries, notably Malawi and Zambia, healthcare systems have already lost a quarter of their personnel to the pandemic. Teachers and students are dying or leaving school, reducing both the quality and efficiency of educational systems. Replacing skilled professionals is now a top priority, especially in low-income countries where governments depend heavily on a small number of policy-makers and managers literally to run the country, particularly its social services.
- There have been steep drops in life expectancy. In four sub-Saharan countries (Botswana, Malawi, Mozambique and Swaziland) life expectancy is now less than 40 years. Were it not for HIV/AIDS, life expectancy in this region would be just over 60 years. In Haiti, life expectancy has dropped from 59 to 53 years.

Having read this wholly depressing selected list of AIDS repercussions (there are many more), you will be asking what can be done by way of either checking the spread of the disease or alleviating some of its worst impacts. Pursuit of that question leads us neatly into the next chapter, and the whole business of healthcare.

Review

10 Try to produce an annotated diagram that traces out the diverse impacts of HIV/AIDS.

11 Discuss these repercussions with your fellow students. Are you able to distinguish between them on the basis of being 'serious' or 'not so serious'?

Enquiry

Visit the UNAIDS website:

http://www.unaids.org/

For one of the global regions other than sub-Saharan Africa, write a brief report (between 500 and 1000 words) summarising:

- the current HIV/AIDS prevalence situation
- the prognosis for the next 10 years
- the main repercussions of the pandemic.

CHAPTER 5

Healthcare provision

The constitution of the World Health Organization (WHO) states that:

The enjoyment of the highest attainable standard of health is one of the fundamental rights of every human being without distinction of race, religion, political, economic or social condition.

So health is a human right, but how are good health and healthcare to be delivered?

SECTION A

Different modes

There are three main ways of responding to the threats posed by disease and ill health:

- **React** – in the *short term*, emergency programmes can meet an urgent, perhaps unseen, need such as an epidemic; while in the *long term*, personnel (doctors, nurses and specialists) must be trained and infrastructure (medical centres and hospitals) provided.
- **Prevent** – immunisation and health education.
- **Ignore** – hope the problems will go away.

Three different levels of healthcare provision are normally recognised:

- **Primary healthcare** is provided in the home, in a clinic or at a health centre. Such care commonly includes basic medical attention from a GP or a nurse attached to a health centre. The services offered include prescribing medication, immunising children and screening for some diseases. They also include dental and ophthalmic care and, in some instances, basic health education programmes. The services are offered locally, since they will be accessed quite frequently.
- **Secondary healthcare** is essentially that offered in hospitals, where patients are admitted for treatment that cannot take place in a health centre. The access route for such care is normally via the primary care system. A doctor refers a patient to hospital for further investigation, diagnosis and treatment (including complex surgery). The secondary sector is therefore more specialised, and will often be less concerned with prevention and more with cure.
- **Tertiary healthcare** is about the delivery of even more specialist investigation and treatment. Typical cases are hospitals that specialise in the diagnosis and treatment of cancer, or undertake heart and transplant surgery.

> **Review**
>
> 1 To what extent do you agree with the view that prevention is the best policy?
>
> 2 Identify the three tiers of healthcare provision in your local area.

But such a classification is not comprehensive. There are other forms that take place outside the medical centre and hospital. Nursing homes for the elderly and hospices for those with terminal illnesses are just two examples. Also to be noted is **alternative medicine**, which has grown rapidly in some Western countries. This includes the services of osteopaths, chiropractors, acupuncturists and homeopaths.

In most countries, it is accepted that health is one of the responsibilities of government. Funding, organisation and the delivery of healthcare are key aspects of that responsibility. Given their different political leanings, governments vary in the way they approach the whole business of healthcare. In most situations, governments have to balance how much of the national budget they spend on health against other demands, such as education, transport and defence (**Chapter 7 Section D**).

SECTION B — National strategies

The aim of this section is simply to illustrate some of the different ways in which healthcare is organised and delivered. Four contrasting national approaches are considered. The USA is chosen as an example of healthcare provision in a free market economy. At the other end of the political spectrum, there are the socialist or communist countries, from whose ranks Cuba is taken as a case study. The UK is selected because of its rather unusual situation of combining a national health service and a market economy. Finally, the case study of Ethiopia is included to illustrate the provision and delivery of healthcare in an LEDC.

USA

Here, the approach to healthcare provision is **anti-collectivist**. The funding comes from:

- Private healthcare insurance schemes. These are arranged by the individual, but are often tied to employment.
- Two state schemes – Medicare and Medicaid. Both were set up in 1965. The former provides insurance cover for people aged 65 and over. The latter covers people on low incomes.

Despite these arrangements, it is estimated that some 33 million Americans are uninsured. They pay for medical treatment on an 'as and when' basis. This is fine as long as the individual's health is good, but can be crippling financially if ill health sets in. The feature of the American system that needs to be stressed is that much of the delivery of healthcare is undertaken for profit. That is as true for individual practitioners as it is for hospital systems that seek profits for their shareholders. In short, healthcare is big business!

UK

The strategy followed in the UK is more **collectivist**. The National Health Service was set up in 1948 to provide healthcare on the basis of need rather than ability to pay. The NHS is funded by general taxation and taxes levied on those in employment (National Insurance). Access to healthcare is usually by registration with a general practitioner (GP), who is responsible for referring patients to secondary healthcare. GPs are paid by the state according to the number of patients registered with them. The NHS is administered by Health Authorities (HAs) – now referred to as 'trusts'. These are given budgets by the government to spend on hospital and community health services. They are also responsible for monitoring the health and the care needs of the populations within their areas. General practices are organised into primary care groups.

The target of much criticism in recent years, the NHS has undergone a raft of reforms aimed at improving the service. Despite this, it is now a burning political issue. It is slowly dawning on the government that throwing ever increasing amounts of public money at the service is not, by itself, going to solve the shortcomings.

Over the past few decades, a private sector has emerged, perhaps as a reaction to growing waiting lists for treatment at NHS hospitals, staff shortages and a general dissatisfaction with the service. There are now private providers, such as BUPA and PPP, which run their own hospitals on the subscriptions paid by members. Most recently, there are plans to involve the private sector in running the NHS. In short, the UK seems to be moving gently towards the anti-collectivist model of the USA.

Cuba

An uprising on this Caribbean island in 1958 led to the establishment of a communist regime, eventually headed by Fidel Castro. One of the major achievements of the Revolution has been healthcare, which is free to every citizen by right. In all of the South, no other country has achieved such remarkable success in such a short period of time. Basic health indicators are head and shoulders above LEDC norms – and in some cases ahead of MEDCs. These achievements are even more remarkable bearing in mind that the country has a per capita GDP figure lower than any other Latin American country, and less than a 20th of that in the USA.

There is a tiered system of healthcare delivery, from '*consultorios*' (small three-storey buildings, where the ground floor is the clinic, the first floor a doctor's flat and the third floor a nurse's flat) to polyclinics, to hospitals and national research institutions. Family doctors and medical services are available from one end of the island to the other. There are 30 000 GPs, roughly the same number as in the UK, but Cuba has only one-fifth of the population. Cuba has 21 medical schools, while the UK has only 12.

Life expectancy for men and women in Cuba today is exactly the same as in the UK. However, there is one major difference between Cuba's health statistics and those of the UK. In the UK healthcare costs £750 per person annually; in Cuba it costs a mere £7. The staggering difference has persuaded the British government to look closely at the Cuban system, to see what lessons might be learnt and applied to the NHS. Three points are of immediate note:

- the Cuban system is patient-centred – this means that patients are represented at every level in the organisation of healthcare
- the quality, dedication and large numbers of family doctors in Cuba mean that much effort can be directed towards disease prevention and early diagnosis
- immunisation is compulsory and the programme covers a wide range of diseases, including meningitis B.

Today, Cuba's healthcare facilities are becoming run down, not because of any fault in the system but, rather, because of the USA's bullying economic blockade of the island. Many basic drugs for the treatment of heart disease, asthma and cancer are no longer available, since purchases from foreign subsidiaries of US drug companies are outlawed. The same applies to basic medical equipment. Sadly, it is the young and the elderly who are suffering most from this wanton outside interference in Cuba's healthcare system. However, there is one positive outcome of this economic adversity. Since food is rationed and meat is scarce, much of the diet is made up of organic fruit and vegetables. Because there is relatively little public or private transport, most people walk or cycle everywhere. Basically, Cubans are much fitter than most!

Ethiopia

Ethiopia is a vast country with a population of just over 60 million. It is also one of the poorest countries in the world. There are under 1500 doctors and 5000 nurses in the entire country. This means that there is one doctor for every 40 000 people, and one nurse for every 14 000. There are nearly 90 hospitals and 260 health centres. The healthcare system provided by the state is seriously challenged by:

- its scarcity
- its inefficient use of resources
- its inaccessibility – the distribution of healthcare is unfair, and nearly a quarter of the health services and over a third of the medical personnel are concentrated in the capital city, Addis Ababa
- the generally low level of health awareness.

There are three outcomes of the inadequate state healthcare system:

- The problem of infectious diseases has gone from bad to worse. Paradoxically, most of the diseases are preventable and curable with minimum inputs, and have been overcome elsewhere in the world.
- A system of private medicine has emerged, but only for the benefit of the relatively small number of rich people. There are now around 200 private clinics.
- Ethiopia has been, and remains, a major recipient of medical aid from both other countries and NGOs. Given that about half the population is Moslem, a significant amount of that aid has come from the oil-rich countries of the Middle East. Much of this aid has been delivered as emergency relief and therefore targeted at the worst areas. As a consequence, only the worst areas have benefited, to the neglect of many other needy areas.

Review

3 Distinguish between **collectivist** and **anti-collectivist** approaches to the provision of healthcare. Which approach do you favour? Give your reasons.

4 Do you think that there should be free healthcare for all, or only for the needy?

5 What lessons do you think that the British NHS might learn from Cuba?

SECTION C

International providers

It is hardly surprising that, no matter where we live on the globe, we should first look to our governments to provide healthcare and to head the war against disease. This point was underlined by the case studies of the previous section. Those case studies also indicated a second source of healthcare, namely the private sector. Figure **5.1** shows, however, that there are other healthcare providers, three of them operating at an international level.

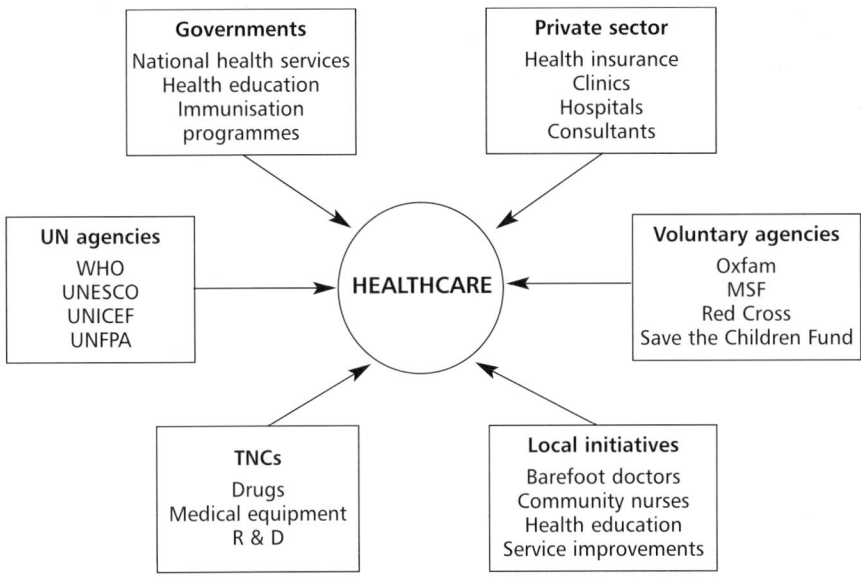

Figure 5.1 Sources of healthcare

Intergovernmental agencies

At the international level, it is the United Nations Organisation that takes the lead, not only in the guise of the World Health Organization (WHO), but also through some of its agencies (**5.2**). All have the promotion of health and welfare as part of their remits.

Figure 5.2 UN agencies concerned with welfare

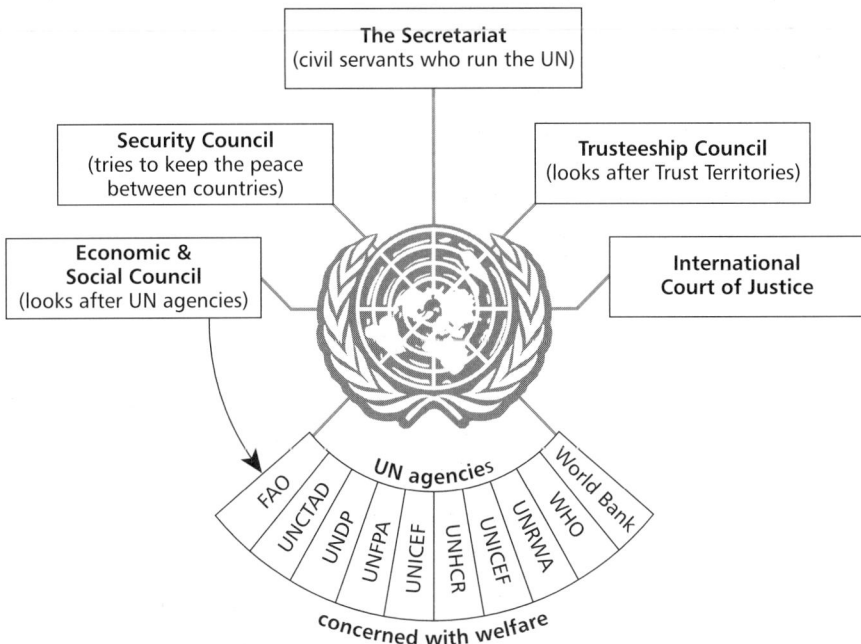

HEALTHCARE PROVISION 57

The World Health Organization (WHO) and the Alma-Ata Conference
The WHO was set up in 1948 by the United Nations Organization (**5.2**). No fewer than 191 states are members. Currently, its main objectives are:

- to help to strengthen national health services around the globe, particularly in LEDCs
- to promote and protect health
- to prevent and control specific health problems
- to support medical and health research.

Perhaps one of the most important events in the 33-year history of the WHO took place in 1978. A conference, jointly organised by the WHO and UNICEF, was held at Alma-Ata (Kazakhstan). It concluded that the health status of millions of people was unacceptable, and it called for a new approach to health and healthcare to shrink the gap between the 'haves' and the 'have nots'. A Declaration on Primary Healthcare launched what became known as the 'Health for all by the Year 2000' strategy. We are now past that target date. Much has been achieved, especially on the eradication of diseases, such as smallpox and polio, but much still needs to be done in terms of extending primary healthcare to poorer parts of the world.

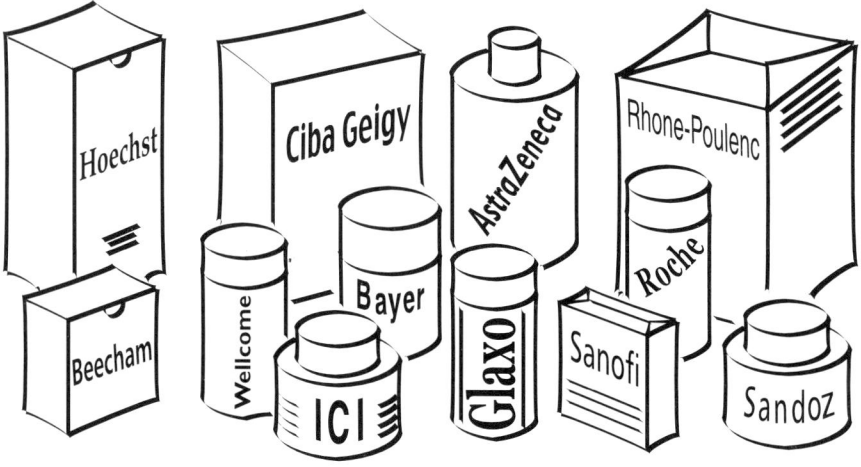

Figure 5.3 Some of the big names in pharmaceuticals

Drugs companies

Many of the world's leading transnational corporations (TNCs) are heavily involved in pharmaceuticals; that is, in the manufacture and marketing of drugs, and in the development of new drug treatments. Some of the more important names are given in **5.3**. In a sense, these companies may be seen as global purveyors of better health. But it is not better health that drives them so much as the huge profits that are to be made from drugs targeted at diseases with high morbidity rates. In LEDCs the 'lucrative' diseases include malaria, measles and TB, whilst in MEDCs they are the treatment of heart disease and cancer. Currently, the race is on to find drugs to combat HIV and AIDS. The company that wins this race stands to make an amazing fortune.

In most MEDCs, the prescription and use of drugs is carefully controlled, usually by government-imposed regulations. However, in many LEDCs the situation is far from satisfactory. Contributors to this unhappy state of affairs include:

- heavy sales pressure by the drug companies, particularly at a government level

Figure 5.4 The global pattern of regular access to essential drugs (1997)

- a reluctance by those companies to lower prices to a level that can be afforded by the poorer countries
- irresponsible selling and inappropriate use
- inadequate labelling and inadequate advice about use
- unrestricted access to drugs.

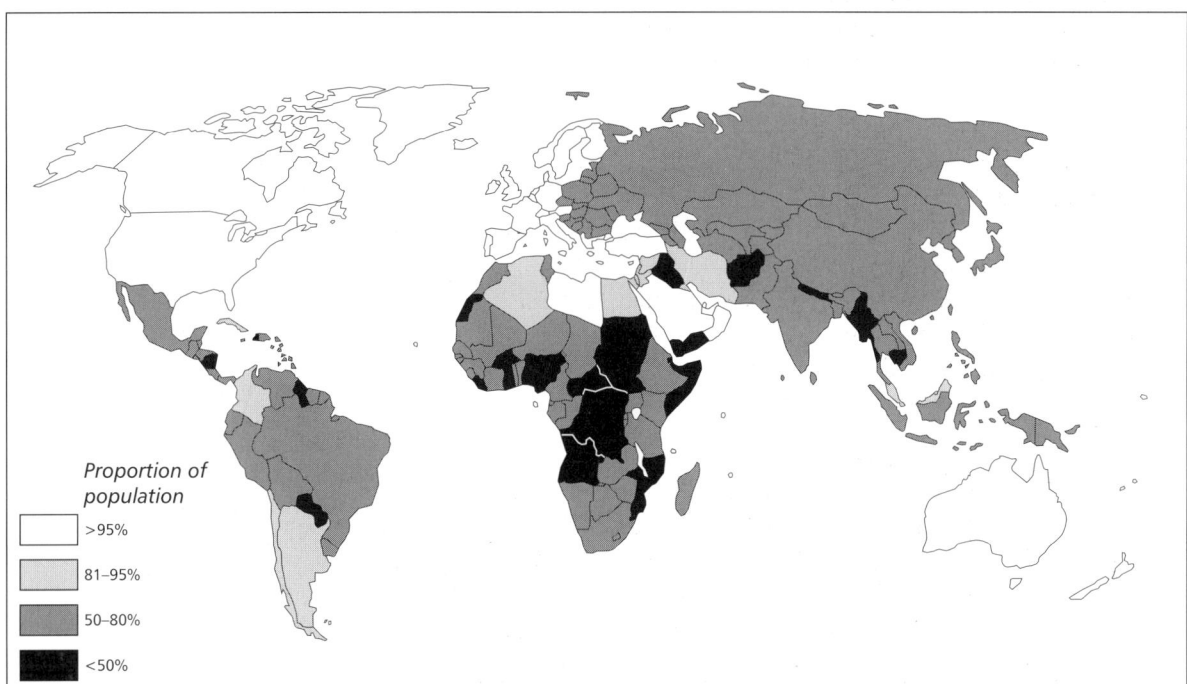

At the time of writing, there is a growing confrontation between US drug companies and countries such as South Africa and Brazil, which have a desperate need for those drugs that can contain the development of HIV. On the one hand, the companies say that every customer must pay the market price. They need to recover their research and development (R & D) and manufacturing costs. The LEDCs argue that they cannot afford the huge costs involved in mounting an effective treatment programme. They ask why the drug companies cannot be more humanitarian and reduce their prices. Figure 5.4 clearly indicates that there are considerable global disparities in terms of regular access to essential drugs. Presumably the cost factor helps to explain the occurrence of the lowest access rates. Even in the UK's NHS, drugs therapies are having to be rationed on the grounds of soaring costs.

Case study: AstraZeneca – an ethical pharmaceutical company

AstraZeneca is one of the world's top five pharmaceutical companies (**5.3**). It is active in more than 100 countries. It has a workforce of over 50 000, who are engaged in R & D, manufacture and marketing of drugs and the supply of healthcare services. Its corporate headquarters are in London; its R & D headquarters are in Sodertalje (Sweden); and it has a strong presence in the key US market. It has six major research centres and manufactures in 19 countries. It spends $8 billion every working day on R & D. Clearly, AstraZeneca is to be seen as a TNC.

Its business is focused on seven important areas of medical need:

- cancer (world number 2)
- cardiovascular diseases
- the central nervous system
- gastro-intestinal infection (world number 1)
- pain control and anaesthesia
- respiratory diseases (world number 4).

Amongst its most recent products are a new treatment for reducing cholesterol levels and an innovative anti-clotting agent for treating potentially fatal blood clots. Alongside these, new treatments are in the process of development for lung disease and a range of cancers.

Voluntary agencies

These are private organisations of a charitable research or educational nature that are concerned with a range of social, economic and environmental issues, of which health is but one. They are also referred to as the **NGOs** (non-governmental organisations). They may act on an international, national or local scale. Some raise money from the public and from governments to help fund healthcare projects in LEDCs or to protect health in disaster situations. Others attempt to educate and campaign on global health issues (such as AIDS) or to lobby governments and international agencies to change public policies.

There are now tens of thousands of charitable agencies worldwide, representing millions of supporters. Amongst the most conspicuous as far as health is concerned are Oxfam, Save the Children Fund, Médecin Sans Frontières (MSF) and the Red Cross.

Review

6 Check that you know the full identities of the UN agencies shown in **5.2** by their initials. You might also refer to the results of work in connection with the Enquiry at the end of **Chapter 1**.

7 AstraZeneca claims to be an 'ethical' company. What do you think this means, and what might be the evidence for it?

8 Visit the website of one of the companies in **5.3** and complete a summary profile like the one for AstraZeneca.

Case study: Médecin Sans Frontières (MSF)

MSF was set up in 1971 by a group of French doctors. It has since grown into an international humanitarian aid organisation that provides emergency medical assistance to populations in need. It has offices in 18 countries and on-going projects in over 80 countries. There are over 2500 volunteers working worldwide and alongside thousands of local personnel.

Normally, MSF collaborates with government authorities, providing assistance with such activities as:

- refurbishing hospitals, clinics and dispensaries
- helping with vaccination programmes
- helping with water and sanitation projects
- working in remote healthcare centres and slum areas
- training local personnel in healthcare matters.

More broadly, MSF is also concerned with drawing wider attention to violations of human rights.

Its current medical activities include the following:

- helping those dying of cold in Moscow
- providing healthcare to the street people of some Brazilian cities
- checking the spread of TB around the Aral Sea
- helping Afghan refugees
- rectifying the catastrophic healthcare situation in Congo.

Review

9. Who should pay for much-needed drugs – the pharmaceutical companies or the consuming countries? Set out the arguments on both sides.

10. Outline the main messages conveyed by **5.4**.

11. Find out more about another of the voluntary agencies that are active in the field of healthcare.

SECTION D — Grass-roots initiatives

The purpose of this section is to make the simple point that there are ways around the two main obstacles that seem to stand in the way of better health in the LEDCs: shortages of public money and trained medical staff. The first two case studies focus on two relatively simple and cheap courses of action at the level of primary healthcare. They may be classified as **bottom-up** approaches to better health.

Case study: Barefoot doctors

The term 'barefoot doctor' was first used to describe a system of medical care established in China under the Communist regime of Chairman Mao Zedong. Men and women with little formal training provide basic medical services and help to educate local communities in preventive healthcare matters such as healthy diet, good hygiene and family planning. The system proved a huge success in China and has been widely imitated since in other LEDCs, where the use of health educators is now quite widespread. Over the past two decades, government-run health services in LEDCs have begun to tap into the rich reservoir of skills found among traditional healers and traditional birth attendants, to help offset the shortage of trained doctors. China has up to 20 times more homeopathic doctors than it has conventionally trained medics. In Africa, there is one traditional healer for every 500 people, compared with one doctor for every 28 000 people.

Case study: The Navrongo project (Ghana)

Gladys Mahama is a community health nurse in northern Ghana. Driving around her 'patch' on a motorbike, she symbolises a health delivery experiment that has the potential to change healthcare arrangements not only in Ghana, but in other LEDCs as well. She is one of 16 nurses who are key workers in the Navrongo Community and Family Planning Project. The aim is to find the best way of delivering health services alongside family planning.

The Navrongo project has shown that a scheme of residential community nurses can be made to work. It has capitalised on experience gained in Bangladesh, so here is an instance of South–South co-operation. Each village in the project area has built a detached hut in which the nurse lives and where she is able to see and treat people, in private, on a one-to-one basis. Thanks to the motorbike, she is also able to visit outlying compounds and the sick who cannot move. Each nurse serves about 3000 people. At the start of the project, only about 1 in 1000 women were using contraception. The figure is now around 1 in 100. Not only has the fertility rate begun to fall, but there has also been a spectacular rise in child immunisation. It now stands at over 85 per cent in some villages, with a corresponding fall in infant and child deaths.

At present, the project is financed by donor money. Those who are able to make a token payment for their treatment are expected to do so. The question now is whether the Ghana government can provide the funds for many more such schemes across the country. Some claim that if projects like Navrongo are able to persuade people to make use of contraceptives, and at the same time improve child survival and the well-being of mothers, then the beneficial effects on national development should ultimately be able to foot the bill.

The next two case studies illustrate two relatively simple steps towards better health but, in comparison, their approach is perhaps rather more **top-down.** They do have cost implications, but the costs are not exorbitant, particularly if they are delivered as key elements in aid packages. They are the sorts of projects that are frequently supported by the voluntary agencies.

Case study: More water – better health

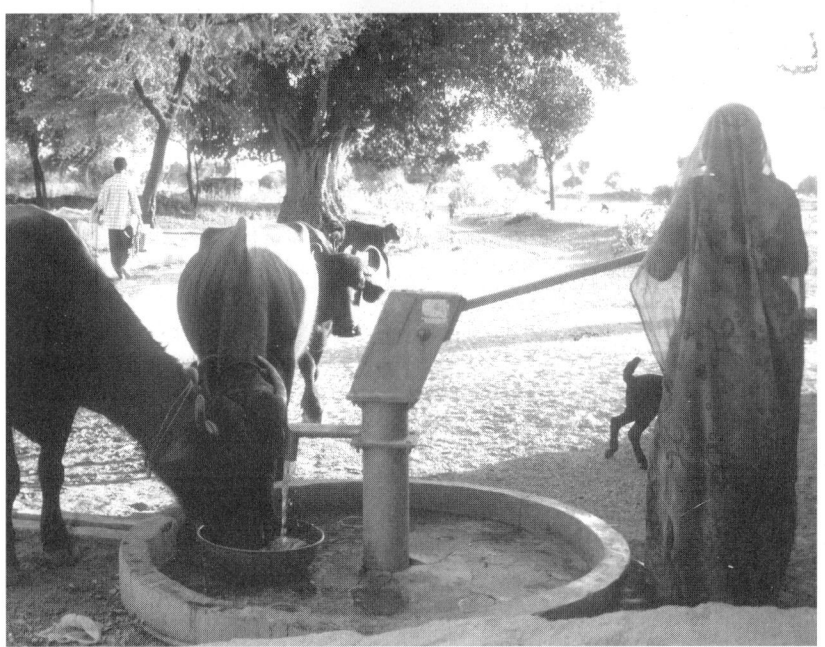

Figure 5.5 An LEDC village well provided by foreign aid

Better hygiene is the key to combating some of the world's worst killer diseases. But how can people living in poverty, who can barely afford soap, be encouraged to be more hygienic? One way is to make water more available to them.

The first lesson of water supply improvement is that those households and communities that will benefit most are those living furthest from existing water sources (5.5). Not only will their health show the greatest improvements, through the reduction of faecal–oral and water-washed skin diseases (see page 30), but they will also benefit most from the saving in time and drudgery (usually the lot of women) spent collecting water from distant sources and carrying it home.

The second lesson is that many poor households are willing to pay for water that is delivered to their door, either by a water-carrier or by pipe. This underlines the point that the time spent collecting water has a money value. That time could be better used doing something that produces income.

The third lesson is that better hygiene lies more in improving the quantity of water that is available than in improving water quality. This is not an easy point to grasp. The fact of the matter is that many of the diseases described as being 'water-borne', such as cholera and typhoid, are passed on not just through water. All of the faecal–oral infections, for example, can also be transmitted by contaminated food, fingers, utensils and even clothes. Clearly, in a situation of improved access to water, a more frequent washing of hands, cloths and utensils can be expected to bring about a considerable reduction in those diseases.

It has been estimated that faecal–oral diseases account for 90 per cent of all the deaths attributed to water-borne diseases and 50 per cent of all hospital admissions. This surely gives an indication of what might be achieved by simply increasing the availability of water. Bringing water closer to people is a much cheaper course of action than improving water treatment.

Case study: Immunisation

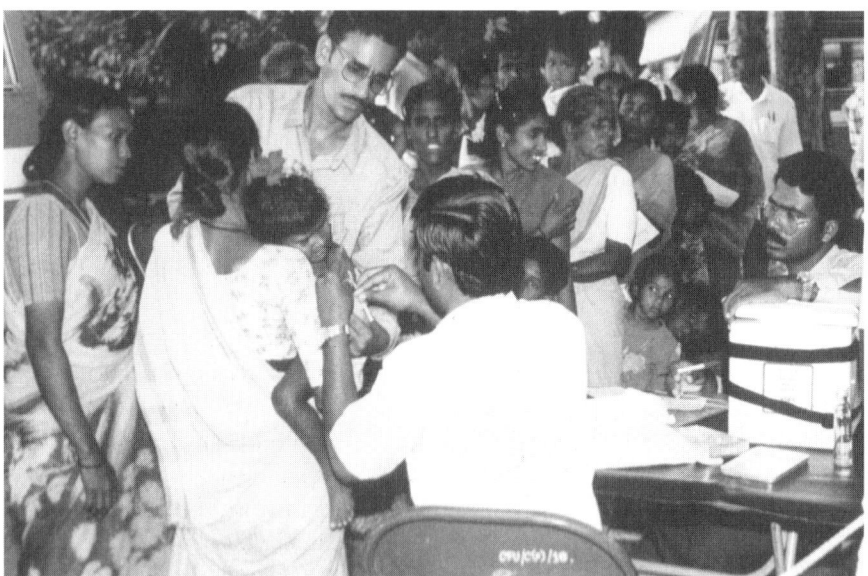

Figure 5.6 LEDC people lining up for vaccination

This is a way of combating disease by creating immunity by artificial means. It can be done by injecting antibodies against specific diseases (passive immunity) or by vaccination (injecting disease-causing micro-organisms to stimulate the body to form its own antibodies without producing the disease) (5.6).

Immunisation against diphtheria, whooping cough, tetanus, measles, TB and polio has saved millions of children from death and disability. Since 1960, child and infant mortality rates have been more than halved by immunisation. In 1980, only 20 per cent of the world's children were protected against the major immunisable diseases. By 2000, the figure had risen to just over 80 per cent. More than 70 LEDCs now report that 80 per cent of all children have been immunised. However, 25 countries (18 of them in Africa) still report coverage of less than 50 per cent for the six major vaccines.

The point about immunisation is that the per capita costs, particularly of the six major vaccines, is quite small. Immunisation is widely accepted as an appropriate form of aid. If the vaccine-producing companies were willing to lower their profits, then immunisation could be expected to contribute even more to the global fight against some of the common killer diseases.

Review

11 What are the important messages of the first two case studies?

12 Explain what is meant by **bottom-up** and **top-down** approaches to healthcare.

13 Assess the relative merits of improved water supply and immunisation as preventive measures.

SECTION E

So who gets what, where and how?

The answer to this multiple question is that much depends on where you are in two respects:

- where you live
- where you are on the affluence scale.

If you live in an MEDC, within reasonable reach of the capital city, and are reasonably well off, then you can expect to access the best possible healthcare, particularly if you are willing to pay. On the other hand, if you are poor and live in a remote part of a LEDC, then perhaps the best you can expect is access to some very basic primary healthcare. The same is probably true of the remote rural peripheries of MEDCs, where high costs and low population thresholds preclude anything more than a minimal provision. Between these two extremes, there is a host of intermediate circumstances. The inequality of access is well illustrated by the percentages of populations with regular access to essential drugs (**5.4**). Over quite large areas of Africa, and scattered parts of South-East Asia and Latin America, less than 50 per cent of people have such access. Over much of the North, with the notable exception of Russia, the access rate is greater than 95 per cent.

Looking at the global situation, what we see is a giant mismatch between the need for healthcare and the degree of provision. This point is graphically illustrated by **5.7**. The first pie chart shows the level of need by global region. The measure used is referred to as the **burden of disease**, and is based on the average number of years of life lost due to premature death and the average number of years spent suffering from disabling diseases. It will be seen that well over half of the disease burden was borne by China, India and sub-Saharan Africa. When it comes to the provision of healthcare, as measured by expenditure in the second pie chart, it will be noted that well over 75 per cent occurs in the established market economies; in other words, in the MEDCs.

Figure 5.7 The global healthcare disparity

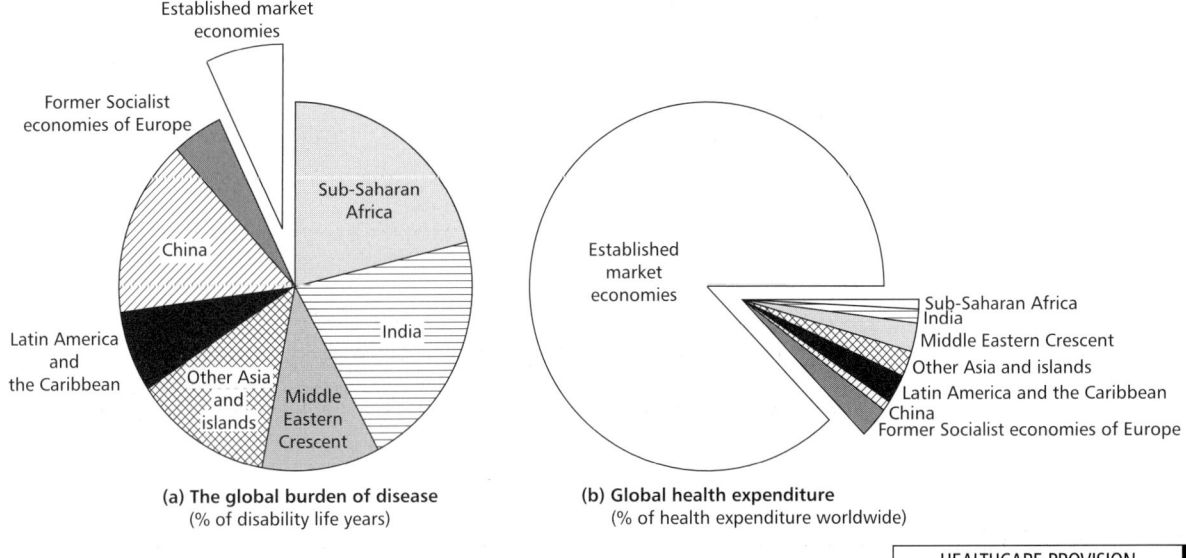

(a) **The global burden of disease**
(% of disability life years)

(b) **Global health expenditure**
(% of health expenditure worldwide)

Review

14 What do you understand by the term **burden of disease**?

15 After poverty, what appears to be the next major obstacle to accessing primary healthcare?

16 How do you explain the fact that access to good healthcare varies even within MEDCs?

Poverty is perhaps the greatest obstacle to reaching healthcare, except possibly in socialist countries, such as Cuba, where access is guided by need rather than by the ability to buy. It is for reasons of poverty that sectors of MEDC society find themselves marginalised and deprived of proper healthcare. This point is illustrated by **5.8**, which shows the distribution of Americans who have no health insurance.

Conversely, there are privileged sectors of LEDC society that are able to access good healthcare either within their own country or by patronising the private health services of other more advanced countries.

If we zoom in still closer, healthcare disparities are revealed even in a prosperous MEDC city such as London. Do the values in **5.9** really suggest that no matter where you live in the capital, you can expect an equal provision of healthcare? Does greater spending necessarily equal better healthcare and access? Might higher levels simply be the outcome of poor organisation and misspending?

To sum up, the minimal requirement of all countries is a system that delivers primary healthcare to all. That care should be not only reactive, but also preventive. Achieving this should be the top priority of the global community, and set alongside programmes of health education. There are some encouraging signs that this might be achievable at a grass-roots level even in the poorest of countries, and in an inexpensive manner. Whether it can ever be achieved at the level of secondary healthcare seems highly unlikely at present, given the inputs of expertise, equipment and money that are required. For the moment, then, let the world concentrate on providing that primary healthcare for everyone. Surely this is a basic human right!

Figure 5.8 The distribution of Americans without health insurance (1997)

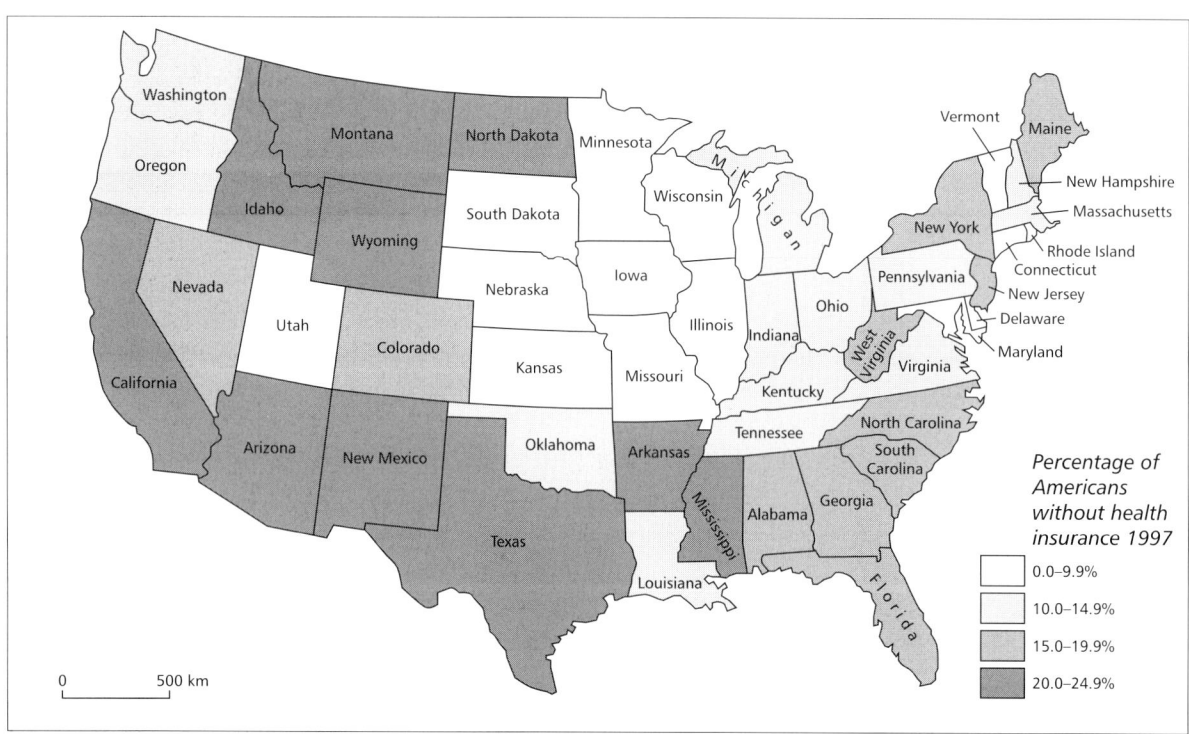

Enquiry

The aim of this enquiry is to investigate the pattern of per capita spending on health services in Greater London.

a Plot the data in **5.9** on the outline map provided (**5.10**), using the choropleth technique.

b Justify the way in which you have categorised the data.

c What other cartographic techniques might you have used to plot the data?

d Describe the pattern shown by your completed map.

e Suggest possible reasons for the difference in per capita spending on health.

f How does your map compare with **6.11**?

Health authority	Per capita spending on health services, 2000–2001 (£)
Barking and Havering	773.42
Barnet, Enfield and Haringey	
Barnet	959.87
Enfield and Haringey	817.53
Brent and Harrow	823.29
Bromley	971.74
Camden and Islington	1067.88
Croydon	925.44
Ealing, Hammersmith and Hounslow	826.21
East London and the City	889.91
Hillingdon	753.76
Kensington, Chelsea and Westminster	1011.24
Kingston and Richmond	829.50
Lambeth, Southwark and Lewisham	886.88
Merton, Sutton and Wandsworth	882.91
Redbridge and Waltham Forest	901.60

Figure 5.9 Public spending on health in Greater London

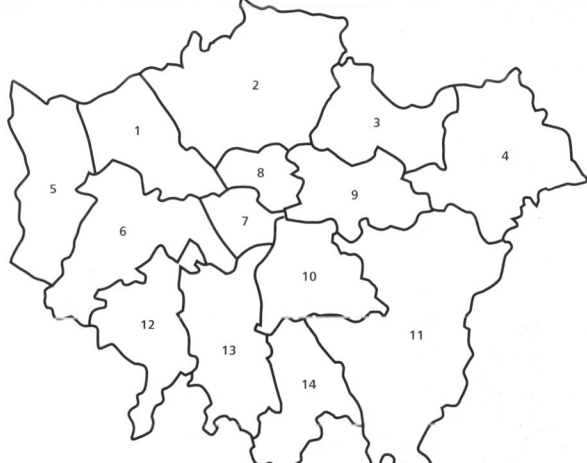

Key
1 Brent and Harrow
2 Barnet, Enfield and Haringey
3 Redbridge and Waltham Forest
4 Barking and Havering
5 Hillingdon
6 Ealing, Hammersmith and Hounslow
7 Kensington, Chelsea and Westminster
8 Camden and Islington
9 East London and the City
10 Lambeth, Southwark and Lewisham
11 Bexley, Bromley and Greenwich
12 Kingston and Richmond
13 Merton, Sutton and Wandsworth
14 Croydon

Figure 5.10 An outline map of the health authority areas in Greater London

HEALTHCARE PROVISION

CHAPTER 6

A wider view of welfare

Whilst most people recognise that health is the single most important component of welfare, it must also be stressed that welfare is a multi-stranded condition. The latter point was briefly illustrated in **Chapter 1** (**Section C**), but it is now explored in more detail, along with another concept introduced in that chapter (**Section E**), namely that of **human security**. Human security is unravelled by UNDP into seven strands (**1.8**). In this chapter, those strands have been reworked a little to define four major dimensions of welfare – medical, environmental, economic and social. The first of these has been thoroughly investigated in the four previous chapters, so let us now focus on the remaining three. An added aim will be to demonstrate that disparities in welfare exist at different spatial scales.

SECTION A — The environmental dimension

Figure **3.1** has already shown some of the potential relationships between environmental exposure situations and specific health conditions. Air and water quality are certainly key elements with respect to disease (see **3.2** and **3.4**), but they also have wider welfare implications. For example, a general sense of well-being is enhanced by being able to wash or bath daily. Rotting garbage and open sewers are offensive to the senses and readily detract from environmental quality and enjoyment, as does air pollution. Two other aspects of the environment, climate and soils, have a direct bearing on another dimension of welfare, namely food security (**Section B**). Climate, on its own, has significant repercussions in terms of housing.

Housing

Housing is included under this environmental heading if only because home is the part of the Earth's space in which we spend much of our lives. It is because of this that housing also has an important bearing on welfare. It is to be regretted, however, that there are few meaningful indicators of the global housing situation. The percentages of dwellings served by water, sewerage and electricity are widely used measures, but they tell us little about housing quantity and quality (**6.1**). Of course, what constitutes adequate housing varies greatly from place to place, particularly between different climatic regimes. For example, a dwelling in the Tropics needs to offer shelter against heat, rain and occasionally high winds. For this reason, it does not have to be a particularly substantial structure. It does not necessarily take much time and money to construct. Contrast this with the housing requirements of high-latitude climates. Here, there is need for altogether greater protection, particularly from the cold.

Homelessness

Poor housing is one thing, but homelessness is another – it is the very antithesis of human security. Homelessness is very much an urban problem, but it would be wrong to suppose that it only occurs in LEDCs. Indeed, the proportion of people who are sleeping rough or in a night shelter may be higher in some of the world's wealthier cities. This is because such cities have a higher proportion of people who lack the income to secure even the cheapest accommodation.

Homelessness is a clear indication that society has failed to provide – for the most needy – the most basic of human needs. The homeless are the victims of the frequent mismatch of housing supply and demand. The global homeless population is currently put at between 100 million and 1 billion – it depends how you define 'homelessness'. The lower estimate probably applies to those who have no shelter at all, and who sleep outside on pavements, in doorways, in parks and under bridges. The higher figure would include those in very insecure or temporary accommodation, much of which is of poor quality.

Case study: Shelter and England's homeless

Shelter is a national campaigning charity set up in the UK to help homeless and badly housed people. It believes that 'Everyone should be able to live in a decent and secure home that they can afford, within a mixed neighbourhood where people feel safe, can work and fulfil their potential.'

Statistics released at the end of 2001 showed there were over 170 000 homeless households in England, amounting to around 410 000 individuals. Of these, nearly half were living in temporary accommodation provided by local authorities – an all-time high. Of these, over 12 000 were housed in bed-and-breakfast accommodation, and of these two-thirds lived in London.

These figures do not include what are called the 'street homeless'; namely, the hard core who sleep out in the open on city streets. A recent government statement claimed that the number of such people had dropped to 600. There are few who believe the claim, but certainly pressure has been put on the street homeless to make full use of hostels run by charities such as Shelter.

Built environment

Nearly half of the world's population now lives in towns and cities. For these people, it is as much the quality of the built environment in general as it is of housing in particular that impacts on welfare and the quality of everyday life. Housing and access to basic services are important parameters of that built environment, but there are others, including:

- traffic congestion
- noise
- pollution
- open space for recreational use
- services – schools, clinics, shops and so on.

Figure 6.1 Built environment indicators for selected cities with populations of between 1 and 2 million

City	% of households with access to				House price to income ratio	Travel time to work (min)
	Potable water	Sewerage link	Electricity	Telephone		
Amman (Jordan)	98	81	99	62	6.1	25
Belgrade (Serbia)	95	86	100	86	13.5	72
Douala (Cameroon)	34	1	95	9	13.4	40
Kuwait City (Kuwait)	100	98	100	98	6.5	10
Omsk (Russia)	87	87	100	41	3.9	43
Phnom Penh (Cambodia)	45	75	76	40	13.4	40
Quito (Ecuador)	85	70	96	55	2.4	33
Rosario (Argentina)	98	67	93	76	5.7	22
Santa Cruz (Bolivia)	53	33	98	59	29.3	29
Tripoli (Libya)	97	90	99	6	0.8	20

The data in **6.1** give some indication of the quality of the urban environment and of urban life in a selection of cities. The cities are all of roughly the same size and are located in countries well down the global league table of development. The penultimate column illustrates one of the particular drawbacks of urban living, namely the expense of housing. The down side is that meeting housing needs deflects household income away from acquiring those other things that are perceived as contributing to welfare (see the **Disposable income** subsection on page 73).

An important point about the built environment is that it is expected to perform basic functions such as providing shelter, safety and access. These, in their turn, become sources of satisfaction and well-being among residents. Built environments can be engineered in ways to improve social interaction, a sense of belonging, personal security and access. Furthermore, there are some who believe that the built environment, through its design and quality, can affect human behaviour in predictable ways. For example, the high incidence of convicted criminals on some council estates in British cities is linked to the **alienation** caused by poor housing and a lack of community amenities.

Case study: Street dwellers in Calcutta

Review

1 Check that you understand what is meant by the terms **quality of life**, **well-being** and **deprivation**.

2 Can you suggest any more measures that might be used to assess the quality of the built environment?

3 How would you rate the quality of life of an Indian pavement dweller? What would you identify as the positives?

Pavement dwellers can be found in most large cities in India. In Mumbai (Bombay) alone there are over a quarter of a million of them. Pavement dwellers live in small shacks made of salvaged materials, which are built against the walls or fences that separate permanent buildings from the pavement and street outside.

Most pavement dwellings are less than 5 m^2 in extent. For this reason, the pavement in front becomes an important part of the domestic space. Water is obtained from nearby housing, whilst use is made of nearby public toilets, for which a nominal payment has to be made.

Pavement households usually have at least one employed member. Contrary to popular belief, very few of these people make their livelihood from begging. Rather, they represent a pool of very cheap labour that is prepared to take on the unpleasant jobs shunned by organised labour. Most work is within the formal economy, as petty traders and hawkers, cobblers and tailors, handcart pullers and waste-pickers. Because they have minimal housing and travel costs, these workers are able to survive on very low wages.

People who become pavement dwellers do so in the belief that it is only a temporary measure. The sad fact is that most never manage to break out of the cycle of poverty and move into better housing.

A WIDER VIEW OF WELFARE

SECTION B

The economic dimension

The three components considered in this section – food, disposable income and unemployment – are all linked to the world of work and subsistence (that is, the means of supporting survival).

Food

Food is the key to survival – without it, we starve. In the context of welfare, there are three issues:

- having sufficient food for survival
- eating the right kind of food
- being confident about tomorrow's food supply.

The first and last of these, taken together, underlie what is referred to as **food security**. This may be defined as the ability of a household, or a nation, to guarantee an adequate supply of food for all – not just today, but also tomorrow. The second has a particular bearing on health. Eating too little of the right food can lead to conditions of **malnutrition**; whilst eating too much (**overnutrition**), particularly of the wrong kind of food, can lead to obesity and all manner of chronic diseases.

There are two routes to obtaining food, both at an individual and a national level. You either produce it yourself or you acquire it from producers elsewhere, by payment, barter or trade. There are few good measures of the adequacy or otherwise of food supplies other than daily calorie intake or the morbidity rates of diseases linked to diet. With regard to the former, it is estimated the average daily requirement for people is about 2500 calories (**6.2**). Most people in the MEDCs of the North receive over

Figure 6.2 The global pattern of daily calorie intake

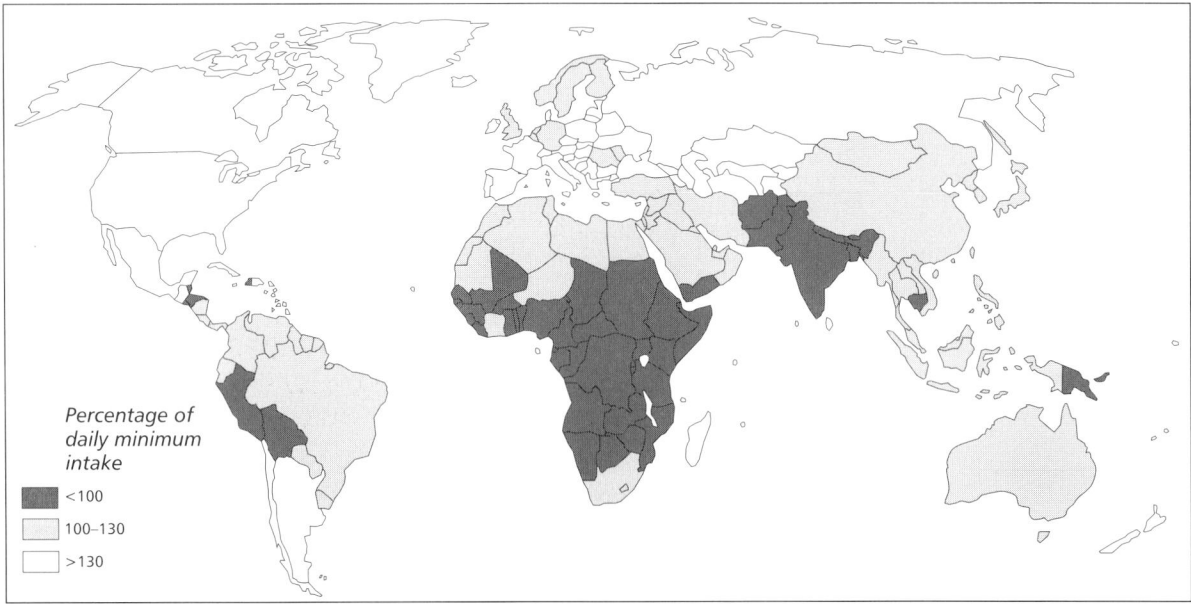

30 per cent more than they need, whilst the average person in the South consumes 10 per cent less than is needed. An intake of less than 1500 calories is likely to result in severe malnutrition. It is also estimated that, today, nearly 600 million people are seriously undernourished.

Remember, when looking at **6.2**, that a country's mean value is bound to conceal extreme values. When it comes to health and welfare, it is those extreme values in which we are most interested.

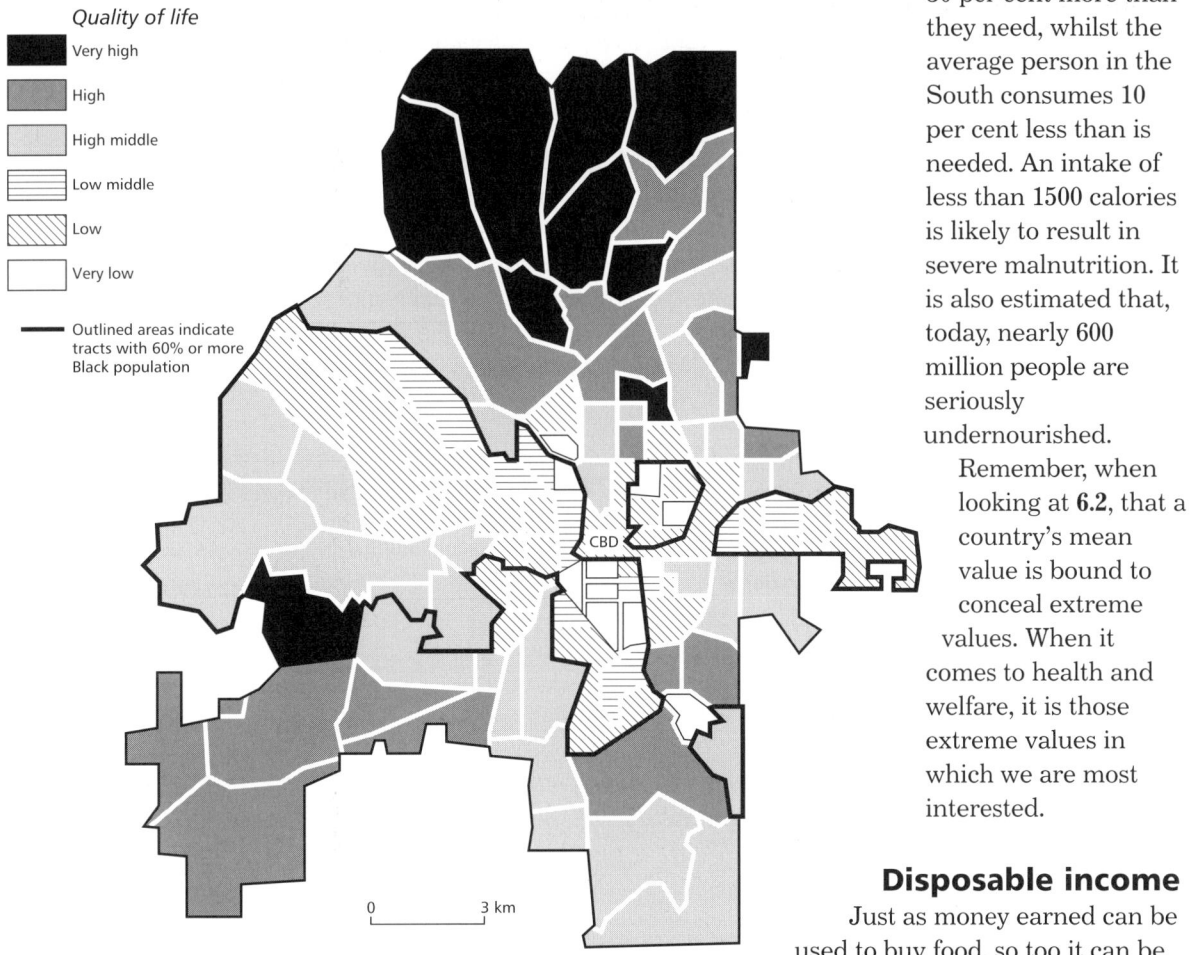

Figure 6.3 Variations in the quality of life in Atlanta, Georgia, USA

Disposable income

Just as money earned can be used to buy food, so too it can be used to acquire those things that we as individuals believe are important to our welfare and well-being. Particularly significant here is what is termed **disposable income**, the amount of personal income that is left after all direct taxes (such as income tax) have been deducted from gross income. For both the individual and the economy as a whole, this gives a measure of the amount of income available for expenditure on consumption, as well as for investment and saving. Thus disposable income provides a pathway to improved welfare and well-being.

Unfortunately, data on disposable income are rarely available. We may expect this to vary from place to place at the whole range of scales from the global to local. In all cases, if it is to have any meaning and significance, disposable income needs to be related to the prevailing costs of living. Perhaps a map such as **6.3** gives an indication of the outcome of disposable income, namely quality of life. In this case, a multivariate measure has taken into account not just family income, but also access to quality housing and good healthcare, as well as population density and law and order.

Unemployment and poverty

Whilst disposable income provides the key to material welfare, the lack of it can so easily lead into a downward spiral of poverty and low levels of welfare (**6.4**). Unemployment probably provides one of the quickest entry points into the cycle of poverty and deprivation.

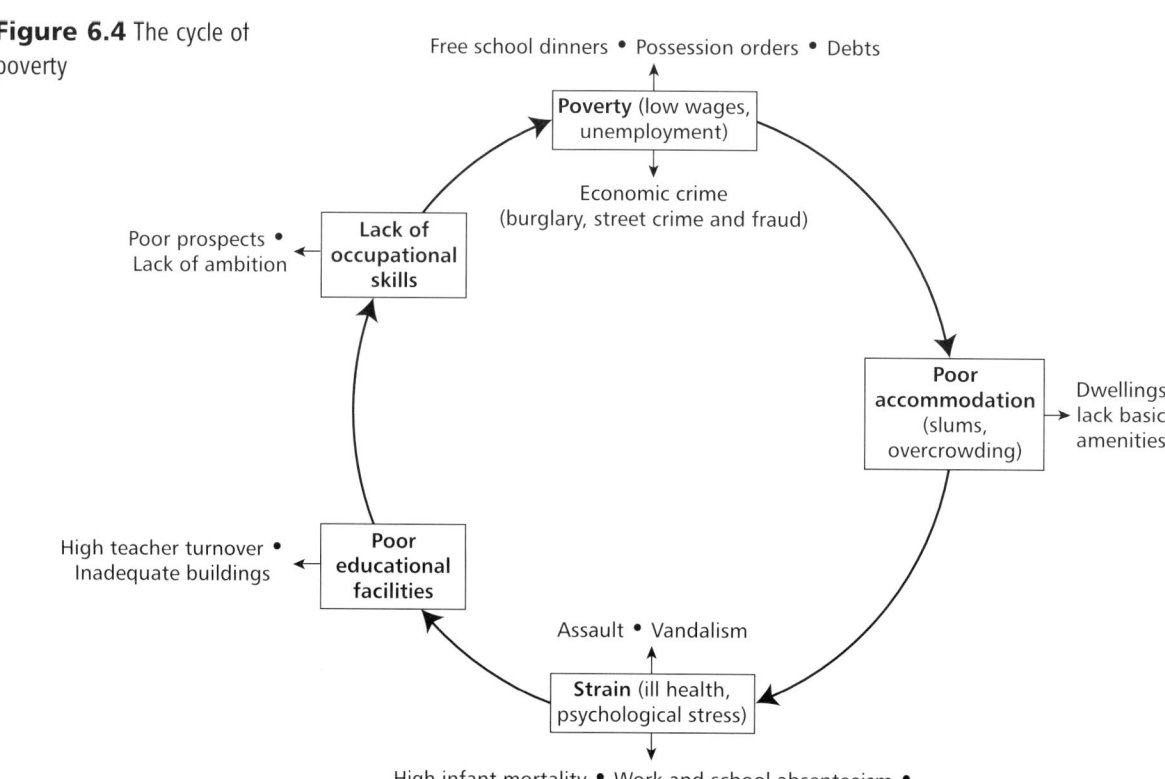

Figure 6.4 The cycle of poverty

At a national level, **6.5** does not show a very close correlation between unemployment and poverty. The suspicion is that the use of aggregate data conceals the existence of pockets of both. Certainly, the data in **6.6** points to the greater prevalence of poverty in rural areas in all but two of the countries. Also revealed are the considerable differences in poverty levels between countries, which – for the most part – are grouped as low-income.

Figure 6.5 The relationship between unemployment and poverty in selected countries

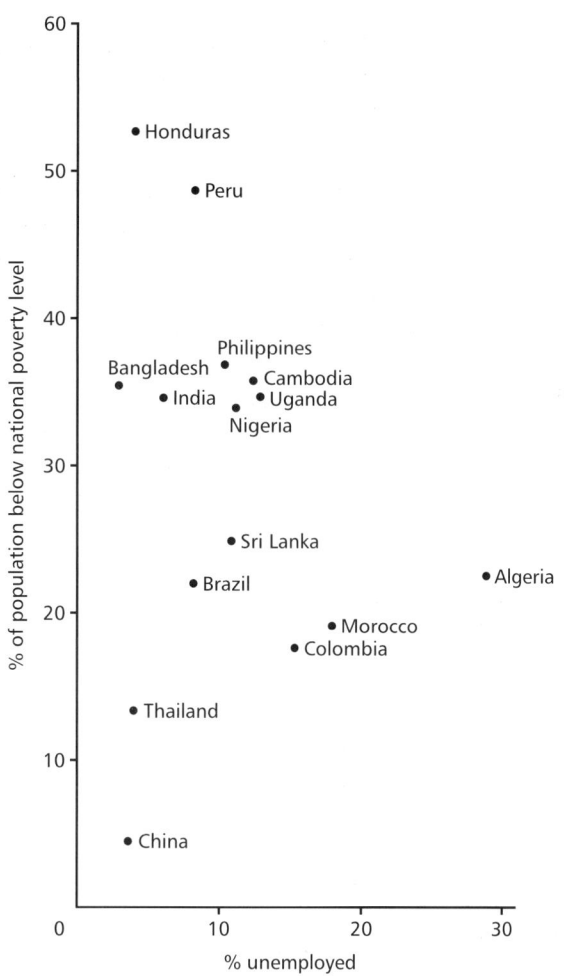

Review

4 Identify the main diseases related to poor diet.

5 Why do you think that poverty levels are generally higher in rural areas than in urban areas?

6 Identify the most extreme anomalies on **6.5** and suggest reasons for them.

Figure 6.6 Rural and urban poverty in selected countries

Country	% of population below national poverty line		
	Rural	Urban	National
Algeria	30.3	14.7	22.6
Bangladesh	39.8	14.3	35.6
Brazil	51.4	13.7	22.0
Cambodia	40.1	21.1	36.1
China	4.6	2.0	4.6
Colombia	31.2	8.0	17.7
Honduras	51.0	57.0	53.0
India	36.7	30.5	35.0
Morocco	27.2	12.0	19.0
Nigeria	36.4	30.4	34.1
Peru	64.7	40.4	49.0
Philippines	50.7	21.5	36.8
Sri Lanka	27.0	15.0	25.0
Thailand	15.5	10.2	13.1
Uganda	10.3	39.1	35.2

SECTION C

The social dimension

In this section, as in the previous ones, the aim is simply to illustrate the different strands and disparities that make up what we might term the 'social dimension' of welfare. By 'social', we mean those aspects that relate to life in organised communities.

Literacy and education

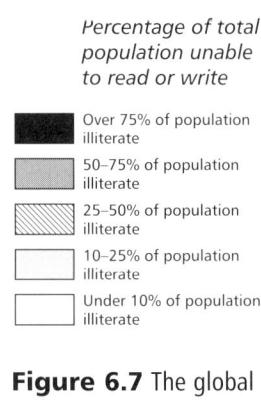
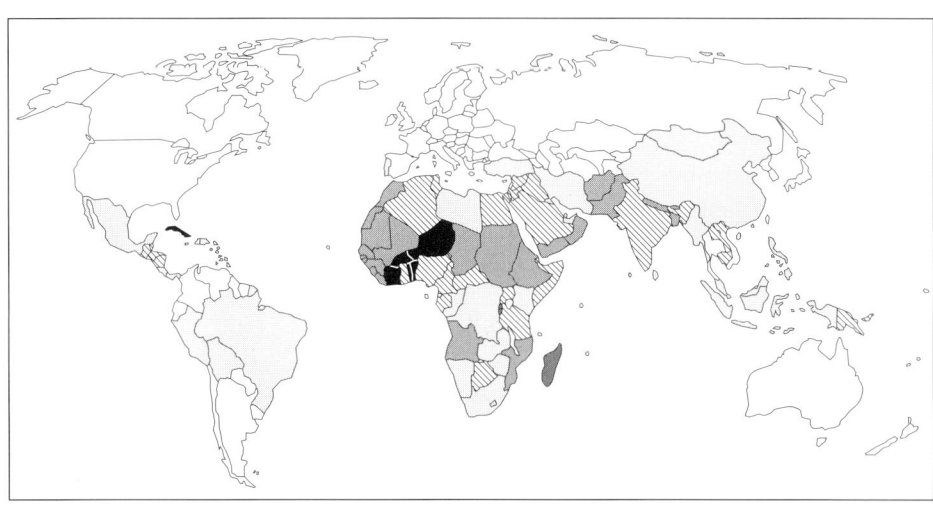

Figure 6.7 The global pattern of illiteracy and education (1995)

The global map shown in **6.7** certainly reveals 'two worlds': across much of Africa, the Middle East and South Asia, over half of the population is illiterate. In those same areas, we find too many countries where compulsory education for children amounts to less than 6 years. Being denied education is perhaps one of the most serious deprivations of all. Without education, the chances of a person advancing in society are substantially reduced. Education, or rather the lack of it, is a key component of the cycle of poverty (**6.4**).

Any nation that deprives its citizens of even the most basic education is unlikely to make much progress along the development pathway. The brutal fact, illustrated by **6.8**, is that in many parts of the world girls are deprived of equal access to basic education. In those areas where education has cost implications, and where domestic incomes are small and access to education has to be prioritised, the practice is to

Figure 6.8 Adult illiteracy and years of schooling in selected countries

Country	Adult illiteracy rate		Expected years of schooling	
	Male	Female	Male	Female
Algeria	9	23	11	10
Bangladesh	48	71	6	4
Botswana	26	21	10	11
Bulgaria	1	2	12	12
Cuba	3	4	12	13
Indonesia	9	19	10	10
Laos	37	68	9	7
Lesotho	28	7	9	10
Mozambique	41	72	4	3
Saudi Arabia	17	34	10	9

give preference to male children. The view is that boys need education to obtain work, whilst girls can contribute by working in the home and eventually be 'sold off' in marriage (see the case study in **Section E**).

Crime

In the present discussion, crime may be seen in two different ways. On the one hand, it may be seen as a symptom that all is not well in society. At the same time, crime is clearly something that can have highly negative impact on well-being and personal security. It is crimes against the person and property that are particularly telling. This covers crimes such as theft, mugging, violence and the threat of it, as well as the mindless vandalism and hooliganism that mark the behaviour of some of today's teenagers. These sorts of crime tend to be at their worse in urban areas. A neighbourhood with a high crime rate, or with a high incidence of criminals amongst its residents, is hardly likely to prove attractive.

Figure 6.9 Street crime hot spots in London

Case study: Suburban nightmare

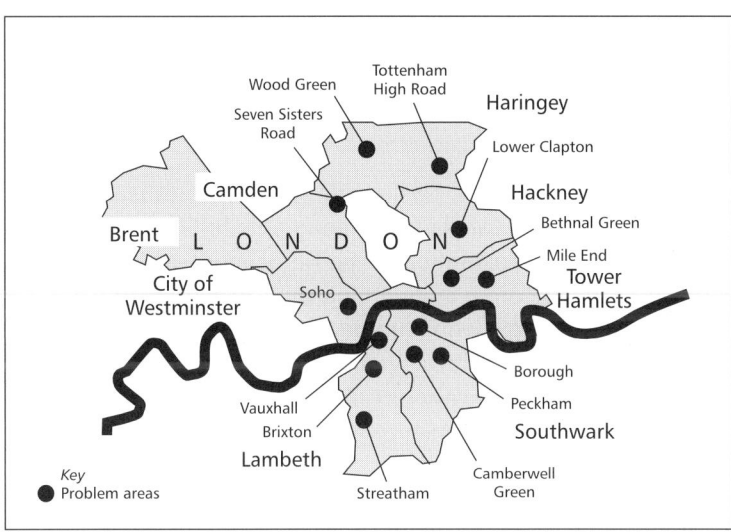

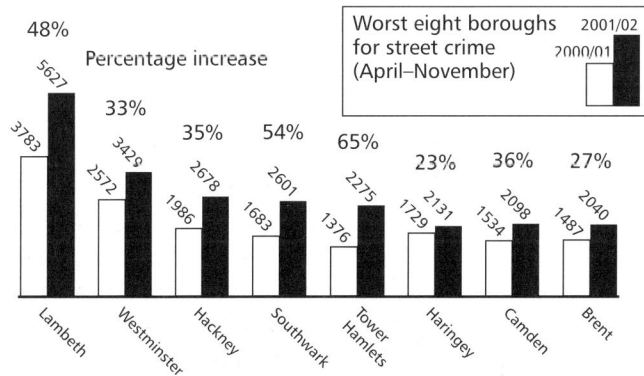

Twice in a week, the unassuming borough of Harrow in north London found itself in the news, but for two very different, but related, reasons. Residents recently opened their Sunday newspapers to find that Harrow is number 13 in the national league table of where millionaires choose to live. But Harrow also appeared high in another league table – as suffering from one of the worst crime waves in the whole of London. Since the 11 September 2001 attacks on the USA, street crime in the borough has increased by more than 100 per cent.

Bad though the situation in Harrow has become, the present street crime rate there does not compare with that in the worst eight boroughs in London (6.9). It is in Inner London that the situation has reached crisis point. In some boroughs, already high rates of crime increased by over 30 per cent during 2001.

The explanation for this sudden and dramatic rise in crimes, such as mugging and the theft of mobile phones, lies in the fact that many police officers have been re-deployed to anti-terrorism duties in Central London and at other strategic targets, With fewer police officers on the beat, petty criminals have seized the opportunity. But, of course, such crime has deeper roots, as for example in the juxtaposition of acute poverty and overt affluence, and in the addiction to alcohol and drugs that makes some people so desperate for the next fix.

Case study: Globalisation and crime

Globalisation creates new and exciting opportunities, and amongst those keen to take advantage are the world's criminals:

- Free movement of capital is something advocated by those involved in foreign investment. But the removal of currency controls means that conditions are ideal for money laundering. The banks of Eastern Europe and parts of the Mediterranean have become important transfer points in the flow of 'dirty' money.
- Lower barriers to international trade and easy transit of goods across national borders are reckoned to be positive developments. But they also mean that a luxury car stolen in Paris can soon reappear for sale in Moscow.
- A greater freedom of movement, particularly of labour, means that it is relatively easy to ship illegal Bangladeshi immigrants to England, or Ukrainian girls to a life of prostitution in the Netherlands.
- The breakdown of the old order in emerging markets has created a growing underclass of people who are ripe for exploitation by the 'crime multinationals' (the organised crime syndicates). The unemployed of South Africa's townships make easy recruits for criminal gangs. In turn, these gangs have helped to make South Africa a major transhipment point in the worldwide drug trade.
- New technology can be exploited for illegal ends: computer hackers can access the confidential accounts held by banks, or 'steal' music, films and software.
- Just as the TNCs have taken advantage of globalisation, so too have the crime multinationals been quick to exploit it. The Chinese Triads are to be found in the restaurant trade in London. The Sicilian Mafia sells heroin in New York, while the Japanese Yakusa are financing pornography in the Netherlands.

Clearly, the control of organised crime must rank high on the global agenda. Failure to do so may be expected to have an adverse impact on the security and well-being of the world's great store of decent, law-abiding people. Any country or government mired by organised crime is likely to find itself missing out on the legitimate benefits of globalisation.

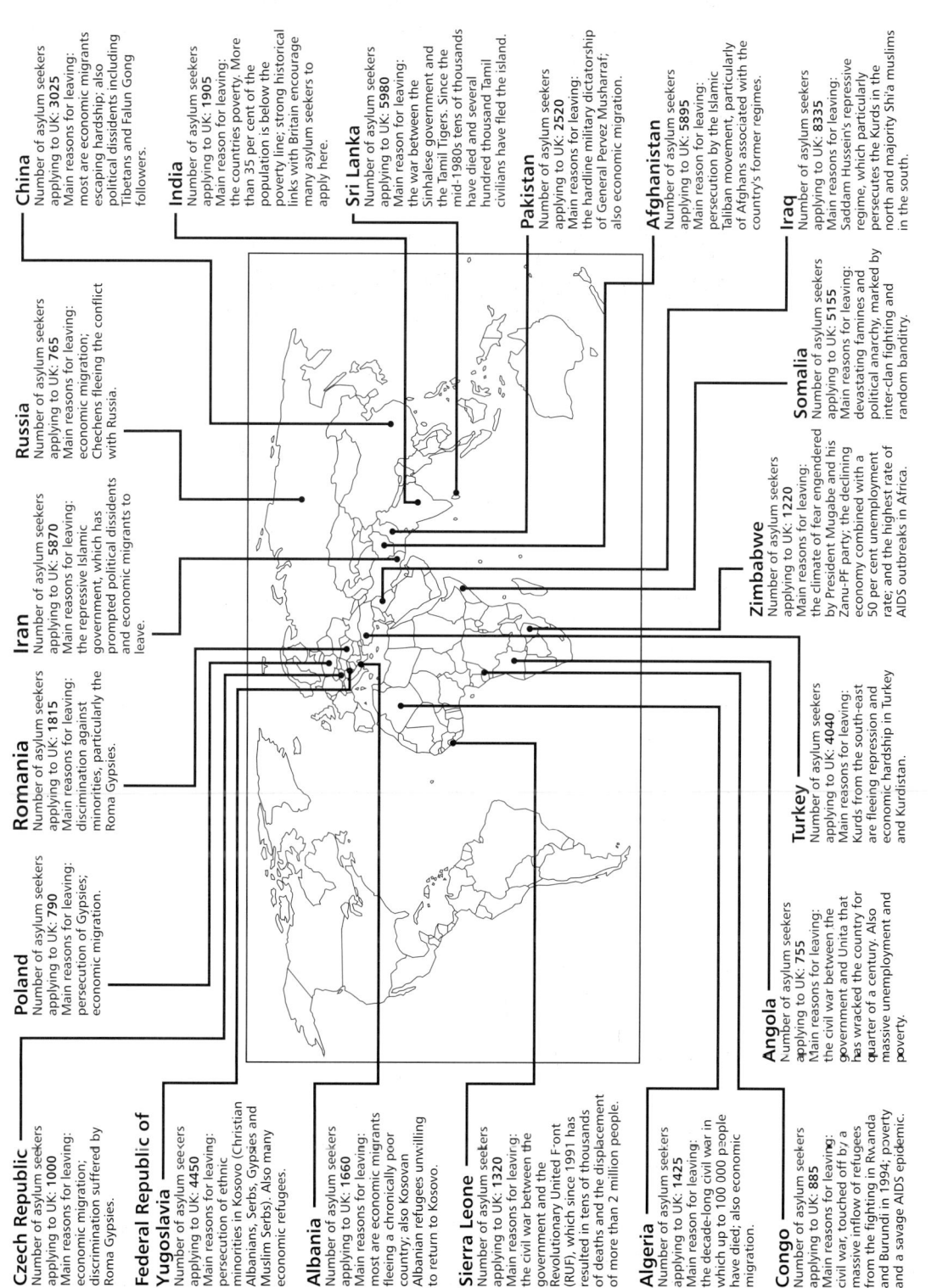

Figure 6.10 Asylum roads to the UK

Human rights

The UN Declaration of Human Rights, adopted in 1948, states that all people have a right to:

- life, liberty and education
- freedom of movement, religion, association and information
- nationality and to equality before the law
- freedom from discrimination and oppression
- equal opportunities
- a sense of belonging
- democratic government.

In today's world, we know full well that such rights are being highly abused. In Zimbabwe, the corrupt and dictatorial regime of President Mugabe has not only abused the economy into bankruptcy, but it is currently suppressing all forms of opposition in a desperate attempt to cling to power. On a wider canvas, the world has never before witnessed such huge volumes of people seeking political asylum. They are driven to do so by feelings of insecurity engendered by persecution and discrimination. At the present time, countries such as Afghanistan, Iraq and the former Yugoslavia are major contributors to the swollen flows of refugees. Potential reception countries within the EU are being inundated by applications for political asylum. The problem for the governments involved is to discriminate between the bona fide asylum seeker and the opportunist seeking personal betterment. The map showing the origins of asylum seekers in the UK (**6.10**) flags up countries where the human rights situation may well be less than satisfactory.

No-go areas

Freedom of movement between countries is regarded by many as a fundamental human right. Presumably that right should also apply to movement within a country. In the UK, however, as elsewhere around the world, that right is being undermined. The threat of crime and the fear of violent ethnic discrimination are deterring increasing numbers of people from either living in or indeed even entering some parts of our cities. No-go areas are more than just perceptions in the minds of people; they are becoming a grim reality. Some of the worse instances arise from the residential segregation of different ethnic groups. For example, Catholics fear to walk the streets of the Protestant parts of Belfast, and vice versa. White people tend to avoid those parts of Bradford in which the Asian community is mainly concentrated. Equally, members of the Asian community feel vulnerable outside those districts. But the problems are not just in the UK. The Black ghettos of US cities have long been no-go areas for Whites.

The point to be made is a simple one. No-go areas are a symptom of personal security under threat. When and where personal security is threatened, so too are welfare and well-being.

Review

7 Argue the case for education being held as the key link in the cycle of poverty (**6.4**).

8 Write a short analytical account based on **6.8**.

9 Identify the various ways in which crime impacts on welfare.

10 Do you think that an increasing level of crime against people and property is more damaging to human welfare than the globalisation of crime?

11 Can you think of any more examples of no-go areas, both in the UK and elsewhere? What are the reasons for them?

SECTION D

Multiple deprivation and its vicious cycles

A vital feature of welfare is the close interconnection of its different strands that have been illustrated in previous sections (plus health, of course). There are recurrent associations, as for example between unemployment, crime and illiteracy (**6.4**) or between poor housing, pollution and disease. People or areas deprived in one way are frequently found to be deprived on a number of other counts. There may indeed be some causal links within these associations, as for example between poor education, unemployment and poverty. Thus, investigations of welfare today often make reference to the concept of multiple deprivation. **Multiple deprivation** refers to an area's, or a group of people's, disadvantage in terms of a range of environmental, economic and social indicators.

A research team at the University of Oxford has devised an Index of Multiple Deprivation (IMD). It takes into account six different 'domains' of welfare:

- income (25 per cent)
- employment (25 per cent)
- health deprivation and disability (15 per cent)
- education skills and training (15 per cent)
- housing (10 per cent)
- geographical access to services (10 per cent).

The percentage figures in parentheses indicate the weighting given to each of the six domains in arriving at an overall IMD.

Figure 6.11 The spatial pattern of multiple deprivation in Greater London (2000)

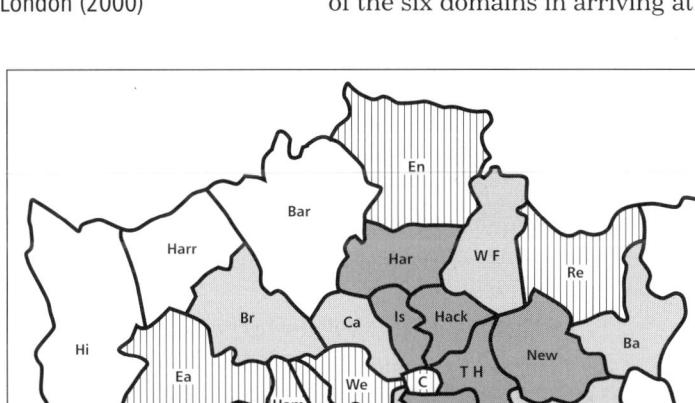

Key
Ba Barking and Dagenham
Bar Barnet
Be Bexley
Br Brent
Bro Bromley
C Corporation of the City of London
Ca Camden
Cr Croydon
Ea Ealing
En Enfield
Gr Greenwich
Hack Hackney
Ham Hammersmith and Fulham
Har Haringey
Harr Harrow
Hav Havering
Hi Hillingdon
Ho Hounslow
Is Islington
K&C Kensington and Chelsea
Ki Kingston Upon Thames
La Lambeth
Le Lewisham
Me Merton
New Newham
Re Redbridge
Ri Richmond Upon Thames
So Southwark
Su Sutton
T H Tower Hamlets
W F Waltham Forest
Wa Wandsworth
We Westminster

Index of Multiple Deprivation score

Worst — 40 and over
30–39
20–29
Best — Less than 20

A WIDER VIEW OF WELFARE 81

In **6.11**, the IMD has been plotted at a ward level. Values range from 57.31 in Hackney (in the East End of London) to 8.30 in Richmond-upon-Thames (in the south-west suburbs). The highest levels of deprivation are found in a triangular area lying mainly to the east of the City of London, with the wards of Haringey, Southwark and Newham forming the apices. Significant limbs of relatively high deprivation are seen reaching to the west (Camden and Brent), to the north (Waltham Forest) and to the east (Barking and Dagenham). Given the weighting of the domains, the map highlights areas of low income, high unemployment and poor health – in a word, poverty. Many of the people who live in these high-scoring areas are victims of the self-perpetuating **cycle of poverty** (**6.4**). Many are held in the so-called **poverty trap**.

Over the years, many theories have been put forward to explain the occurrence of poverty and deprivation:

- **Structural class conflict theory** argues that poverty and deprivation arise out of the way in which society organises itself. Inequality is in-built and perpetuated by the social system.
- **Institutional management theory** blames governments and private institutions (such as banks and building societies) and their inability, or unwillingness, to allocate resources, goods and services in a fair way. There is an inherent bias that favours the rich. Words such as 'disadvantaged' and 'underprivileged' are commonly used.
- **Cycle of deprivation theory** reasons that children born into deprived households and into deprived areas have fewer opportunities to improve their lot. They are therefore trapped in a vicious cycle from which it is extremely difficult to break out. Individual progress is inevitably retarded.
- **Culture of poverty theory** puts the emphasis on individual inadequacies and on a general sense of failure that becomes deeply engrained in some households and families. In such domestic environments, aspirations are never more than low. There is a rather fatalistic attitude to low achievement.

It would be wrong to see these four theories as being in any way in competition. The truth of the matter is that the causes of poverty and deprivation are rooted in all four. Having said that, it is also fair to say that the last two theories find particular favour today, whereas 20 years ago it was the first two that were backed more strongly.

Review

12 What do you understand by the term **multiple deprivation**?

13 Which of the four theories appeals to you most? Give your reasons.

SECTION E

Meeting needs

There are three aspects to be considered here: **need**, **provision** and **access** (**6.12**). We are already aware that need varies greatly from place to place; that is, in terms of what is specifically required and to what degree. What has to be done to ensure that general well-being reaches a satisfactory level? With regard to provision, the key questions are 'Who provides?' and 'What is provided where?' In an ideal world, few would disagree that access should be based on need and that there should be equality of access. In reality, problems are created by the ability and willingness of people to pay for what they need. So to what extent should access be conditioned by affluence? Then, there is the geographical impossibility of providing services that are equally accessible from all parts of a country. Depending on how these issues are resolved, disparities in welfare may increase or decrease.

We instinctively think that it is the responsibility of government (national, regional and local) to provide for welfare needs. But even a government that sets out with the best intentions can only do what its public funds permit. If the country or region is poor in resources, undeveloped and its population earns little, then there is a very slim chance that much, if anything, can be done to meet welfare needs. Here we encounter, once again, that vicious disparity or mismatch between level of need and the ability to meet needs. The only way in which a country or region is going to break out of the downward spiral created by that inverse relationship is by seeking help from outside, or by discovering grass-roots solutions that are effective but inexpensive – that rely on ingenuity rather than on vast sums of money.

Figure 6.12 Meeting needs – key questions

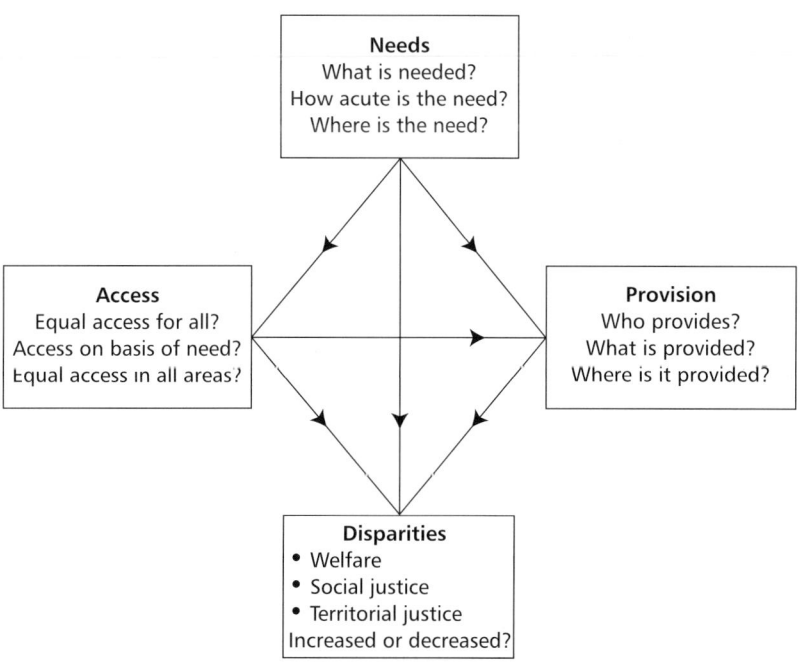

Another grim reality is that even where a general provision for welfare needs is made, rarely is there equal access. No matter at what spatial scale – national, regional or local – there are always people who are in some way marginalised. They are denied access to what should be theirs as of right. Such marginalisation is widespread even in the most affluent countries of the world. Indeed, the general level of wealth accentuates the existence of these pockets of poverty and deprivation. Such pockets also exist even in socialist states.

Contributory benefits	Non-contributory benefits
Incapacity benefit	Child benefit
Jobseeker's allowance	Disability living allowance
Maternity allowance and leave	Housing benefit
Retirement pension	Income support
Sick pay	Invalid-care allowance
Widow's benefit	Working families tax credit

Figure 6.13 Some components of the UK's welfare safety net

In some countries, attempts are made redress welfare disparities by providing various forms of social benefit. 'Aid' of the sort shown in **6.13** might be seen as forming a kind of welfare safety net. Hopefully it catches most of those who, for whatever reason, are unable to provide adequately for themselves. The UK's scheme of social benefits may not be particularly generous. Undoubtedly, there are countries that make better provision for the really needy. Equally, there are many countries that do even less, even to the point of doing nothing at all.

SECTION F

Ways forward

This discussion of welfare concludes with three case studies. Each relates to a different dimension of welfare. Each shows the sort of thing that can be done to improve welfare at a grass-roots level and, in particular, to draw in those who are so often marginalised.

Case study: Site and service schemes

Site and service schemes are an interesting attempt that is being made in a number of LEDCs to improve the living conditions of the urban poor. They have been applied to some of the older squatter or shanty areas of cities as far apart as Lusaka (Zambia), Rio de Janeiro (Brazil) and Jakarta (Indonesia). They begin with the city authorities recognising the rights of the squatters to the land that they occupy. Relatively small amounts of public money are then spent on providing a basic infrastructure of water and electricity supplies, roads and waste disposal. In return, the squatters are expected to improve their homes by replacing the scrap building materials with bricks, mortar and proper roofing, and possibly adding properly built new rooms.

Public investment in the physical infrastructure is perhaps the key. One immediate benefit is more hygienic living conditions. A lessening of disease improves the prospects of obtaining and retaining a job. Work, in turn, means the money to improve both housing and diet. A virtuous upward spiral is initiated.

With increasing numbers of people flocking to LEDC cities, the site and service schemes promise reasonably healthy living conditions. Outside the cities, permaculture promises a sustainable food supply.

Case study: Permaculture

Food security is one the most basic of all the different components of welfare. In those parts of the world where this security is threatened by a shortfall in food, it makes sense to make the best possible use of what the natural world provides. Permaculture (permanent culture) does just this. The system uses no external inputs, such as chemicals and pesticides. Each part of the farm system benefits other parts of the same system. For example, tree crops are grown. Whilst those trees tap soil moisture, their leaves enrich the soil and help the growth of vegetable and cereal crops between the trees. The trees also provide shade. Indigenous trees are preferred, for part of the technique involves making insecticide sprays from their leaves, bark and wood. Small numbers of livestock are kept and these provide both food and manure for working back into the soil. The soil is heavily mulched to keep it cool and damp; it is never left exposed to the sun and wind.

There is little new in permaculture; it capitalises on what has been known for generations. Its simply brings together what we might call 'best practices' into a single farming package. Permaculture is knowledge-intensive, so training is needed. There are now well over 100 training centres in the LEDCs. The system can be adapted to work well in both humid and arid tropical environments. In most cases, farmers can expect to increase their yields from upwards of four times within a few years. Besides delivering food security to holders of relatively small parcels of land, it allows farmers to reduce the proportion of the land used for immediate subsistence needs. Thus the opportunity arises to raise a cash crop or two. The only costs involved in the system are those of training and providing advice.

While having a roof over your head and enough to eat promise survival, the pathway to a better tomorrow lies in education. And ensuring that girls have the same access to education as boys promises well not just for half the population, but for society as a whole.

Case study: Educating girls

It is well substantiated that women and girls are treated as second-class citizens in many parts of the world – uneducated, neglected and abused, invisible and undervalued. It is also widely acknowledged that educating girls is the single most important step that governments can take to improve the health and welfare of their citizens.

Educated women marry later
- fewer children
- greater economic independence
- more experience of life outside the home

Educated women practise family planning
- family size adjusted to available resources
- more say in decisions about family size
- reduced fertility and population growth

Educated women have healthier children
- better hygiene in the home
- more informed about diet
- more likely to have children immunised and to attend antenatal clinics

Educated women raise 'better' children
- more awareness of the social and psychological needs of children
- more awareness of the rights of children
- more ambitious for children to 'get on'

Educated women are more confident
- higher level of expectation, particularly from services
- greater say in family decisions
- more likely to challenge traditional views about gender roles and discrimination

Educated women are more productive
- greater likelihood of adopting improved farming methods, farming being the traditional duty of women in many LEDCs
- greater participation in the labour force
- higher rates of pay

The bottom line to all this is that it only requires three things:

- a guarantee of equal access to education
- a modest increase in the proportion of public funds allocated to primary and secondary education
- a change in traditional views about gender

to bring about an upward spiral of widening benefits.

Whilst the basic message of this chapter has been a rather depressing one, it is perhaps right to try to end it on a positive note. Hopefully, you will agree that these last case studies do offer the prospect of improved well-being for many who currently desperately need it.

Review

13 Explain what is meant by the terms **access** and **marginalised** in welfare studies.

14 Sketch the virtuous upward spiral started by site and service schemes.

15 Does permaculture have any drawbacks?

16 Can you think of any other beneficial spin-offs from ensuring that girls have equal access to education?

Enquiry

1. Access the website:

   http://www.detr.gov.uk

   and extract Index of Multiple Deprivation data for the wards of an area known to you. Produce a map like **6.11**. Does the pattern show anything that conflicts with what you previously thought about the area?

2. Investigate the welfare situation in one of the countries shown in **6.10** as contributing to the volume of UK asylum seekers. Produce a report setting out the reasons for the outflow of migrants.

CHAPTER 7

Future threats and challenges

In this last chapter, the aim is simply to outline a selection of welfare issues that, at the time of writing, are thought likely to pose particular threats and challenges in the 21st century (**7.1**). Be warned, though, that the selection is very much a personal one. In many ways, it is hoped that these predictions are wrong, for maybe what you are about to read has more than an air of 'gloom and doom'. It would be easy to say that the threats and challenges lying ahead are the worry of the rising generation that will have to confront them, rather than of the present older generation. A much more responsible comment, however, would be to say that all of us, regardless of age, have an obligation to become:

- better informed about welfare issues
- more concerned about the welfare of others
- more proactive in the correction of welfare disparities.

Failure to move in these directions certainly promises a much less secure future for everyone.

Figure 7.1 Future welfare: threats and challenges

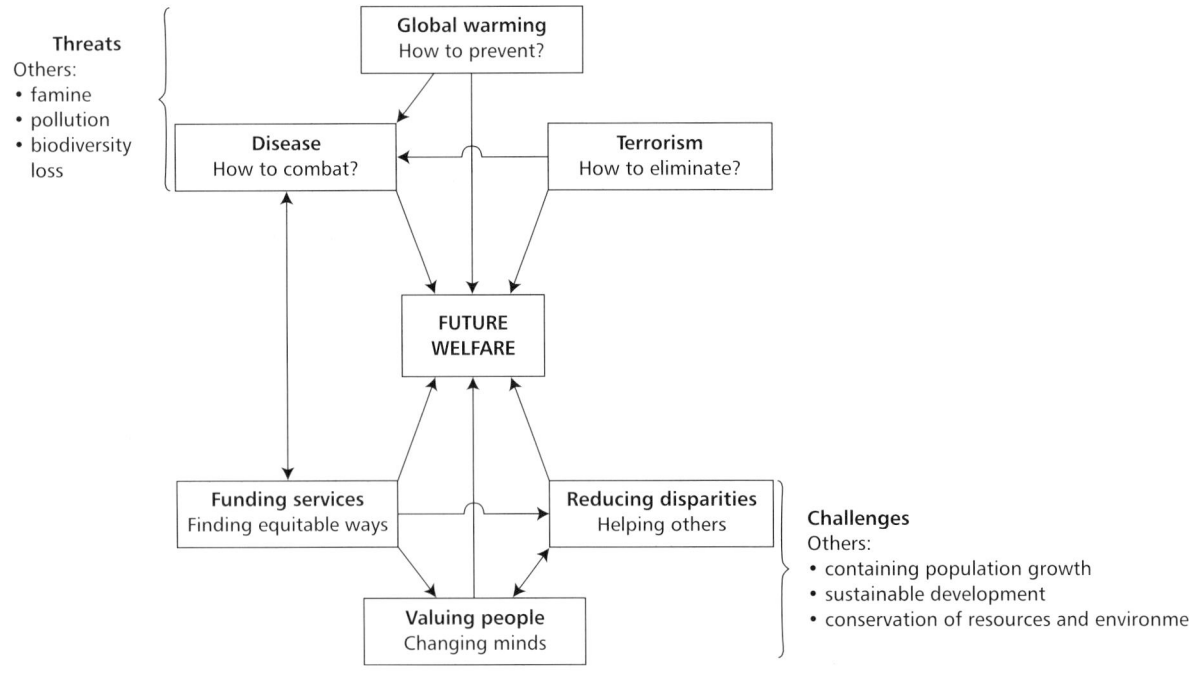

SECTION A

Diseases old and new

The language used in discussing health frequently makes use of the phrase 'the battle against disease' (**7.1**). That battle is an endless one, for a number of reasons:

- There are still many parts of the world where living conditions fall below that necessary to sustain basic good health. The problem is that these regions can act as breeding grounds for diseases that are subsequently transmitted, largely by international travellers, to parts of the world that are supposedly clear of them. Typhoid (see the case study on page 25) and cholera are two such diseases.
- 'Old' diseases that were thought to have been 'conquered', perhaps by vaccination programmes, have a nasty habit of returning, and often in a more vicious form. Frequently, a time lag exists between the identification of a new strain and the production of an appropriate treatment. The resurgence of some old diseases is particularly worrying (see the next case study), and especially where social systems have deteriorated.
- History warns us that 'new' diseases keep popping up at irregular intervals, often taking the medical profession completely by surprise. They vary greatly in the degree to which they threaten people and the time it takes to discover the causes and devise a remedial strategy. The 1996 World Health Organization Report claimed that 30 new diseases had emerged during the previous two decades. Among the new diseases, there are new variant CJD, Legionnaires' disease and Ebola fever, as well as, of course, HIV/AIDS.

In the remainder of this section, the aim is to illustrate the last two of the above bullet points by means of three case studies.

Case study: TB poses a growing threat to global health

Tuberculosis (TB) is an airborne infection spread by coughing. The disease can affect any part of the body, but it is usually sited in the lungs, where it slowly destroys tissue.

TB was rife in Britain in the 19th and early 20th centuries. Rapid industrialisation meant that workers malnourished by poverty were thrown together in appalling housing conditions, thus enabling TB to spread. Thanks to nationwide vaccination programmes and the gradual demolition of slums, the disease has largely disappeared from the UK and many other MEDCs.

Recently, it has been estimated that a third of the world's population carry the disease, but nine out of ten do not show symptoms. It infects one person every four seconds. Eight million people a year develop the disease, of which 3 million die. Many of its victims are young. TB is therefore responsible for more deaths than AIDS or malaria, but combined with HIV it becomes a deadly cocktail. Because HIV reduces immunity, so latent TB infections are increased. As one scientist has put it: 'HIV is to TB what matches are to kindling, and Africa could be just the start of the wildfire ... It is like Ebola with wings.'

Adding to the concern about the spread of TB is the growing incidence of drug-resistant forms of the disease. Normally, the TB bacterium is susceptible to basic antibiotics. However, to eradicate the disease completely in any individual patient requires prolonged medication. Incomplete courses of treatment add to the threat of drug resistance. This is happening in Russia and the epidemic there could provide the basis for a global spread of drug-resistant forms of TB.

Another aspect of the TB threat, particularly in MEDCs, lies in the tendency for GPs to ignore TB as a diagnosis, for three reasons:

- the misplaced belief that TB has been eradicated
- an unfamiliarity with the symptoms of the disease
- the lack of a drugs company producing any new and eye-catching treatment that would remind doctors to think of TB when diagnosing.

But the fact of the matter is that TB is making a comeback in the UK. The Borough of Newham in East London has become the 'TB capital of the affluent Western world'. There are now 108 cases of the disease per 100 000 of its population, putting it ahead of Russia, where the collapse of the public health system has led to 91 cases per 100 000. Half of the figures in Newham are a result of people from India, Bangladesh and sub-Saharan Africa seeking asylum. Many of these asylum seekers carry the disease in a harmless latent form. It is the dire housing conditions they face in the UK that stimulates the disease.

In 1998, the WHO organised a meeting of all the leading pharmaceutical companies to explore the possibility of developing an effective TB drug. The companies indicated that it was not worth them developing drugs that would give a profit of less than $350 million over a five-year period. In their view, a TB drug would not meet this requirement!

Case study: The birth of BSE and a new variant of CJD

The immense, and totally justified, publicity given to HIV/AIDS has overshadowed the attention paid to other emerging diseases. Bovine spongiform encephalopathy (BSE), widely known as 'mad cow disease', is one of these. It is an incurable brain condition in cattle, which causes neurological disorders and eventually results in death. It was first discovered in the UK in 1986. It is now thought to have been caused by feeding to livestock a meal derived from the offal of cattle and sheep.

By the time the disease had been diagnosed and a large-scale slaughtering of infected animals had been undertaken, BSE had spread to the livestock herds of several other European countries and the USA. That spread was worrying enough, but still more alarming was that the disease had apparently jumped the species barrier. In the early 1990s, it began appearing in the human population as a new variant of Creutzfeldt–Jakob disease (CJD). This is a fatal degenerative disease that affects nerve cells in the brain, causing dementia and seizures before death. It took a long time to establish the link between BSE and CJD. Its transmission is believed to have been due to the consumption of BSE-infected beef. It had previously been thought that CJD was caused by administering growth hormone, derived from human sources, to under-sized children. Very recently, a possible link has been forged with a polio vaccine, the preparation of which involves the use of cattle material. It is suggested that one or more batches may have used material derived from BSE-infected herds.

There is still much to be learnt about BSE, about the degree to which CJD has entered the human food chain and about expected levels of mortality. At present, concern centres on sheep and whether or not BSE has jumped that particular species barrier. It has been known for a long time that scrapie in sheep and CJD have a similar infective agent. If BSE is already in sheep flocks, then the trail of future CJD fatalities could be immense.

Case study: The global war on AIDS

With HIV/AIDS rising so quickly up the league table of 'big killers', it is exceedingly worrying that, as yet, medical science has been unable to come up with an effective vaccine. The best that has been achieved so far are drugs that slow the progress of the HIV and therefore delay the onset of AIDS.

In June 2001, the UN launched a comprehensive campaign against HIV/AIDS. Each member government agreed to pursue a number of targets that included:

- lowering the infection rate amongst 15–24 year olds by 25 per cent by 2010
- reducing the proportion of infants infected with HIV by 50 per cent by 2010
- improving healthcare for the victims of the disease and increasing access to anti-HIV drugs
- providing a supportive environment for orphans and for HIV-infected children

- taking action against those factors that make people particularly vulnerable to HIV infection, such as poverty, illiteracy, lack of information about self-protection, lack of access to the commodities of self-protection and all types of sexual exploitation of women, girls and boys
- enlisting the help and resources of NGOs and TNCs.

Perhaps one of the difficult challenges is to overcome the complacency that exists both at a personal and a national level. 'HIV will never catch me' is a dangerous way for anyone to think. Equally, governments of countries with low prevalence rates today may well sit back and take a relaxed view of things. However, they could well find a rather different situation tomorrow, particularly if the spread of the disease there is in its early stages. Low national prevalence rates can be very misleading. They often disguise serious epidemics that are initially concentrated in certain localities or among specific groups. Such epidemics can quickly spill over into the wider population.

Review

1. Write a brief account outlining the main ways in which human diseases are spread. Rank those ways in what you think is their order of importance.
2. Outline the factors that are making the spread of TB a growing threat to global health.
3. Find out what the latest position is with regard to BSE and sheep.
4. What are the latest official figures for CJD deaths in the UK?
5. Go through the list of bullet points in the AIDS case study. Are they feasible?

SECTION B

Global warming

The debate about global warming is mainly about causes. There are few who now doubt that global warming is already happening and that it is likely to continue into the foreseeable future (**7.1**). Among a number of growing concerns is the expected impact of this climatic change on human welfare, particularly health.

Amongst the list of direct impacts are those associated with an increased frequency of extreme weather events. More heat waves will lead to a rise in mortality, particularly amongst the very young and the very old (**7.2**). Although it is more difficult to predict the effects of storms and floods, we can be reasonably certain that huge areas of crops and large numbers of people will be wiped out. You need look no further than the delta areas of Bangladesh to imagine the scale of the potential damage and destruction.

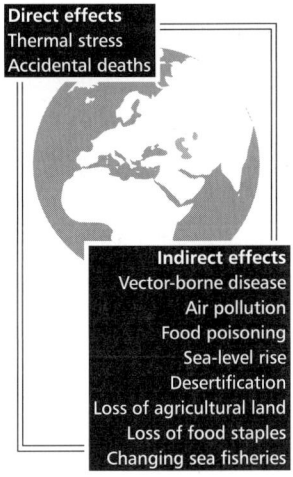

Figure 7.2 Some welfare impacts of global warming

The main indirect effects of global warming include (7.2):

- a 'speeding up' in the spread of infectious diseases
- damage to health due to increased air pollution
- a loss of food security.

An earlier case study (page 32) indicated that malaria has already begun to spread into new territory. The same is true of dengue fever. A temperature rise of 1–2°C could result in an increase of the at-risk population by several hundred million, with 20 000–30 000 more dengue deaths a year by 2050. Increased heat will mean that the incubation of many viruses and bacteria will be accelerated. Extremes of weather are something that favours the rat and its vector capacity to spread disease. Higher levels of pollution are expected to increase the number of deaths due to respiratory diseases.

With regard to food security, it is estimated that 350 million people are already dependent on permanent food aid (7.3). Increasing population densities, shrinking amounts of farmland (due to desertification, coastal erosion and so on) and shifting rainfall patterns are simply raising the risk of even more frequent crop failures. These failures, in their turn, will not only raise mortality rates. They will also trigger large migrations as people search for food security. Such movements will simply add to the strains already being placed on land and food supplies elsewhere.

Figure 7.3 Distributing food aid

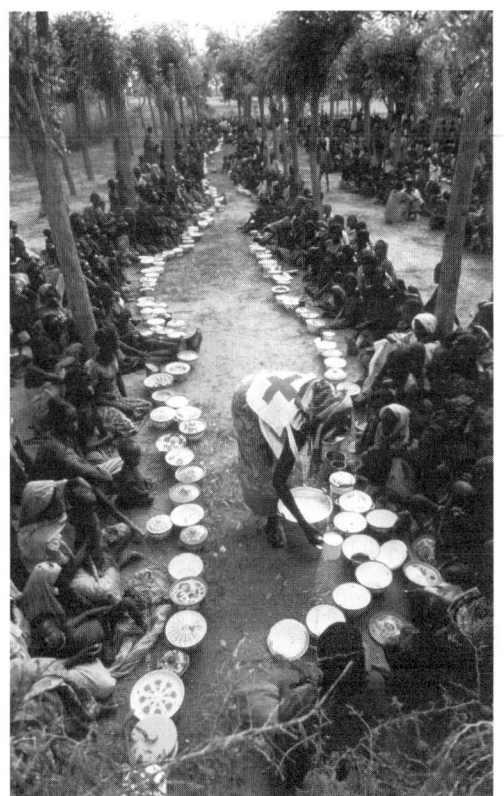

There is a tendency to think that the adverse impacts of global warming will be largely confined to the LEDCs. Mention of rising sea levels usually causes people to think only of low-lying islands in the Pacific and Indian Oceans. But what about the Low Countries of Europe, East Anglia and the very densely populated coastal lowlands of Japan, not to mention the US state of Florida? The risk of the permafrost melting is a less publicised impact. Large buildings and much of the physical infrastructure in permafrost regions could well be seriously damaged. Moreover, permafrost contains large quantities of methane gas. This is a greenhouse gas (GHG), and if it were to be released, global warming would be given a further boost.

In the view of most meteorologists, everything possible needs to be done to prevent global warming. The main way is to bring down GHG emissions. Concerted global action is required – countries must act together. On a per capita basis, the USA uses 10–20 times as much fossil fuel as most LEDCs. But the LEDCs cannot afford the costs of installing GHG-free technologies – not immediately, that is. There has to be **redistribution**. This requires that MEDCs reduce their GHG emissions more and at the same time accept that LEDCs will do less. The EU has already agreed a GHG reduction scheme along these lines, but the USA has not.

Review

6 Explain why global warming is expected to lead to increased air pollution.

7 Can you think of any welfare benefits that global warming might bring?

8 Try to identify the possible welfare costs and benefits to the UK of global warming.

SECTION C

Valuing people

Ageing populations

In all MEDCs fertility is low; in some it has fallen to the point at which deaths now outnumber births. The outcome is a static (in some cases, contracting) and ageing population – a new stage in the Demographic Transition model. By 2025, there will be more than 800 million people aged over 65 in the world. Two-thirds of them will be in the LEDCs. There will be 275 million people over the age of 60 in China alone – more than the total population of the USA today. Increases of up to 300 per cent in the older population are expected in many LEDCs, particularly in Latin America and Asia, within the next 25 years. Population ageing has immense implications for all countries. In the 21st century, one of the biggest challenges is how best to maintain the health, independence and mobility of an ageing population.

Caring about the elderly in MEDCs

In the UK, there are already almost as many people aged over 64 as there are children under the age of 15. For every 100 people of economically active age, there are nearly 30 elderly people. Of course, a fair proportion of these elderly people are fit and financially independent (thanks to personal savings and private pension schemes). But the sad fact is that, at an individual level, fitness (physical and mental) and independence deteriorate with time. For many, there comes a time when independence gives way to a dependence on care. Initially, it may be the family that provides the care, but the care requirement may further increase to the point at which the family can no longer cope. Specialist 'round-the-clock' care is needed. The move to residential care is most often a traumatic event for the elderly, but such a removal can also involve crippling costs. At one time, the expectation in the UK was that the state would meet those costs. That, sadly, is no longer the case. Crudely put, the elderly are expected to pay the bill until their money runs out.

Country	Pension contributors (% of labour force)	Average pension (% of per capita income)
Algeria	31	75
Burundi	3	57
Chile	70	56
Czech Republic	85	37
Egypt	50	45
Greece	88	86
Guatemala	23	28
Jamaica	44	26
Japan	98	34
Jordan	40	144
Switzerland	98	44
Turkey	35	113
UK	90	est. 20
USA	94	33

Figure 7.4 The vulnerability of pensioners in selected countries (1995)

In many countries, care for the elderly is fast becoming a major issue. Many societies expect people to provide for their needs in old age by contributing to state, private or both types of pension scheme. The data in **7.4** are worrying, if only because the percentage of the labour force doing just that is well below 100 per cent in many countries. Not only that, but the pension income is but a fraction of the average earned income. Implied here, therefore, is the expectation of a lower level of welfare and well-being. A drift towards poverty is threatened. It should also be said that there are many countries in which no provision at all is made for old age.

Recently, it has been claimed that the impact of an ageing population on healthcare costs is not now as great as had been thought. Studies have suggested that a quarter of a person's healthcare costs come in the last year of life, and that this remains true no matter at what age they die. Clearly, such a claim is difficult to believe in the case of the increasing number of people suffering from Alzheimer's and other dementia diseases. The mind may be weakened, but physical resilience and care can mean that survival runs into years. Remember, too, that the welfare of the elderly requires more than medical services. As people live longer, so the demand rises for a whole range of specialist care services. These range from purpose-built sheltered accommodation to day centres, from the prescription of glasses and hearing aids to the provision of zimmer frames and wheelchairs, from free travel on public transport to large print books in libraries.

The term **ageism** is now well established in the English language. It refers to increased discrimination against elderly people. In the UK, ageism focuses particularly on those people in their late fifties and sixties. In the world of work, there is a tendency to see such people as ready only for the scrap-heap. They are thought of as being unable to keep up with new technologies and unable to cope with the pressures of the workplace. **Voluntary redundancy** and **early retirement** are the excuses given for laying off older employees. It would seem that some employers place no value at all on experience and the wisdom that comes with age.

Caring for the elderly in LEDCs

What about the elderly in LEDCs? With lower life expectancy, they may be proportionately smaller in number, but they too have welfare needs. Who provides? Traditionally, it has been the extended family, on the basis of the simple principle that children look after their parents. Such an arrangement is helped by the custom for the different generations of a family to live together in the same dwelling or compound. However, that tradition is being shaken by the development process, particularly by urbanisation. A rising volume of rural–urban migration is an integral part of the earlier stages of urbanisation. It is the young and economically active who make up the majority of migrants; the elderly tend to be left behind in the countryside. So there is certainly the problem of looking after these 'abandoned' elderly. Further down the line, there comes a time when these rural–urban migrants themselves become elderly. Who looks after them? It may well be that, as is commonplace in urban communities, the children have moved on to another town or city. The scarcity and cost of urban accommodation may well mean that there is no space for elderly parents. To make the situation more difficult, there is no fall-back in most LEDCs in the form of state welfare. For sure, as life expectancy increases, so caring for the elderly will become an even more pressing issue in LEDCs.

Case study: Traditional care under threat in Tunisia

Less than 5 per cent of Tunisia's 9 million people are aged over 64. Only 800 people live in homes for the elderly. The family is still the bedrock of Tunisian society and virtually all of the country's elderly people are looked after by their children or relatives. Working people are obliged to give their parents a pension. The elderly are respected for their wisdom and experience. The state only steps in to take over responsibility for the relatively few elderly people who have no family to look after them.

Today, however, there are changes that threaten to de-stabilise this family-centred culture. A shortage of work is encouraging more and more people to emigrate. Contact with tourists and foreign media is also helping to persuade people that the grass is greener outside Tunisia. Those emigrating are mainly in the economically active age range. They leave behind their elderly parents, depriving them of the traditional support of a secure home, loving care and often a pension.

Sex discrimination

Whilst ageism is a form of discrimination that is becoming increasingly evident in MEDCs, so discrimination on the basis of sex remains widespread in LEDCs. Women are still treated as second-class citizens. They are deprived of those things that most Western women now take for granted, such as:

- an education
- a chance to seek a life outside the home
- a choice in marriage

- a say in family size
- a chance to live.

Yes, there are still parts of the world where the killing of girl babies is practised. Such is the strength of preference for male heirs!

Case study: The Taleban bans women

The rule of Afghanistan by the Islamic fundamentalist Taleban movement was a particularly bad time for women. During the five-year regime:

- women were only allowed to do housework and cook
- they were forced to wear the burka (a veil that covers the whole body) when outside the home
- they were not allowed to wear 'Western clothes' or make-up at any time
- they were not allowed to talk to men in public
- many were denied medical treatment if they could only be seen by a male doctor (there are precious few women doctors)
- girls were excluded from schools.

Any transgression of these rules was usually punished by a public beating. Mercifully, the Taleban regime has been overthrown, but sadly much of this sort of discrimination prevails in a less extreme form in other parts of the Islamic world.

Much of the business of the Cairo Conference on 'Population and Development' (1994) focused on gender, particularly the status of women in LEDCs. It highlighted the need to abandon traditional gender attitudes and to protect the basic human rights of women. Since then, movement in the right direction has been little and patchy. It does seem incredible in this day and age that so many male-dominated governments fail to see the simple bottom line: a society that deprives half of its population of their rights halves the potential of that society to progress. All societies should value all of their members. In order to achieve this, minds and attitudes that have become deeply entrenched over time will need to be changed radically.

Review

9 What do you think is meant by the term **human resources**?

10 Weigh up the pros and cons of persuading people to retire before the statutory age.

11 Try to explain why in many societies the tradition is:
- to prefer boys to girls
- to treat women as second-class citizens.

SECTION D

Paying for welfare

Virtually all of the different aspects of welfare considered in this book cost money. In many – but certainly not all – MEDCs, people tend to look to their governments to foot the bill. Whilst it might look as if they are doing so, it is public money that the governments are spending; that is, money mainly collected in the form of taxes.

	% of GDP		
	Education	**Health**	**Defence**
High HDI			
Canada (0.932)	7.0	6.9	1.4
USA (0.927)	5.4	6.5	3.6
Japan (0.924)	3.6	5.6	0.1
UK (0.918)	5.4	5.9	3.0
Medium HDI			
Malaysia (0.768)	5.2	1.3	1.4
Romania (0.752)	3.6	3.5	3.5
Brazil (0.739)	5.2	1.9	1.9
Jordan (0.715)	7.3	3.7	8.8
Low HDI			
Nepal (0.463)	3.1	1.2	0.8
Uganda (0.404)	2.6	1.6	3.8
Burundi (0.324)	3.2	1.0	4.9
Ethiopia (0.298)	4.0	1.7	1.8

Figure 7.5 Welfare spending in a sample of countries based on HDI values (1996)

Sharing out the cake

The challenge that faces all governments is to decide how the national income is to be shared amongst a wide range of competitive causes, including welfare in its broadest sense. The inevitable situation is that the demand for money exceeds what is available. Giving more money to one cause usually means depriving another. The task is to balance the books and to produce a budget that fairly reflects the country's priorities. Figure **7.5** shows that combined expenditure on health and education (perhaps the two most important aspects of welfare) rarely exceeds 15 per cent of GDP, even in the most advanced and prosperous countries. In the poorest countries, the combined share rarely exceeds 5 per cent.

Perhaps you might be surprised to see that **7.5** also includes information about defence spending. You might say that defence can hardly be thought of as welfare. But think about it for a moment and remember the concept of human security. For most countries, spending on defence means protecting national security. National security, in its turn, overarches most of the other forms of security that have been discussed in this book.

In LEDCs, governments are far less well placed to pay for their welfare needs. Tax revenues and the level of economic output are low, and this limits the actual amount spent on welfare. Over the years, some help has been available in various forms of aid from better-off donor governments and NGOs. The cruel fact of life is that the expectation of aid is good when the global economy is booming. In recession, however, when the need for help is much greater, the willingness and ability to give that help are much less. Figure **7.6** gives some idea of how much of their national wealth the leading MEDCs 'give' in aid.

What is all too clear today is the failure of governments (not just in the LEDCs) to deliver adequate public services, from clean water to primary schools, from proper waste disposal to health services. In most cases, the reason is inadequate funding. To add to the problem, it is most often the case that those who need those services most are the least able to afford them.

Figure 7.6 National spending on overseas aid (1995)

MEDC	% of GNP
Netherlands	0.76
France	0.64
Canada	0.42
Germany	0.33
UK	0.30
Japan	0.29
Italy	0.20
USA	0.15

Micro-privatisation

This is a term being increasingly heard these days, particularly in NGOs and international development agencies. Basically, it is a process whereby governments agree to hand over responsibility for public services to small private or community enterprises. Pioneering projects around the world are already showing promising results in the form of improved quality, efficiency and access. Still more impressive is that these results have involved significantly reduced costs. The vital principle underlying the projects is a pragmatic one; namely, that those who consume services should pay at least some of the costs, if not all. Such an arrangement is surely preferable where there has been a total failure to provide free services.

Ironically, micro-privatisation is not too far removed from the so-called 'privatisation' of the UK's essential industries and services that took place under the Conservative governments of the 1980s and early 1990s. Amazingly, the principle is now even being pursued by the present 'New Labour' government in its reform of the NHS!

It needs to be pointed out that micro-privatisation also recognises that there will be instances in which the need for welfare is so critical that it simply will not do to rely on the hope that consumers will pay. In such situations, providers need to seek external funding, particular from NGOs and charities. This is well illustrated by the next case study.

Case study: Clinics for prostitutes in Nicaragua

The failure of publicly operated health systems to serve the poorest and most needy is illustrated by the case of female prostitutes. They suffer high rates of sexually transmitted disease (STD), unwanted pregnancy and induced abortion, and are at high risk of developing and transmitting HIV/AIDS. Because of the stigma attached to their profession, prostitutes are typically marginalised by government-run health services. More than most, they require regular health checks and treatment. In general, they are unable to afford the fees charged by private clinics.

The scheme followed in Nicaragua – particularly in the capital city, Managua – has been set up by the Central American Institute of Health (ICAS). It involves issuing prostitutes with vouchers that entitle them to free care from any one of a variety of private, NGO and public clinics. These clinics have been specifically contracted to the scheme, and they provide a high standard of care, but their business is not exclusively to do with the scheme. Regular distributions of vouchers are made in the red-light districts. The prostitute takes a voucher to one of the contracted clinics and receives advice and appropriate treatment. The clinic returns the voucher to the agency and is reimbursed the agreed fee per

Review

12 How would you prioritise the allocation of public funds to defence, education and health? Justify your ranking of the three demands.

13 Outline the arguments for and against the welfare services principle that 'the user pays'.

treatment. The whole scheme is run by ICAS. The government is not directly involved, but it does contribute to the funding. Most of the money comes from NGOs and charities, including the Elton John Foundation.

The scheme has been up and running since 1996. It is extremely difficult to assess the proportion of prostitutes who are participating in the scheme. There is a high turnover in the profession, as the average career of a prostitute is only about two years. It is equally difficult and too early to know to what extent the scheme has contributed to a lowering of HIV transmission. Nonetheless, the voucher system has proved to be an effective way of targeting health resources at a marginalised, impoverished and needy group. That so many of the women have used the vouchers suggests that the model might be used to target other groups of people or particular areas in dire need of welfare help – people and areas that so often escape the welfare safety net.

SECTION E

Reducing welfare disparities

Much of the content of this book has revealed the existence of 'two worlds' involving both places and people. They are variously described as 'the rich and the poor', or as 'the haves and the have nots'. The adjectives do not matter that much. What does matter, for example, is that place disparities exist mainly at two scales – within nations and between nations. The challenge ahead is to reduce those disparities and close the so-called **development gap** (**7.1**). Figure **7.7** sets out a minimal agenda for moving in that direction; it comprises seven specific actions.

- **Fair trade** The needs of MEDCs and LEDCs are to a degree reciprocal – each has much of what the other needs. There is a great potential for interdependence and trade. Unhappily, the prevailing situation has been one wherein the strong exploit the weak. The conditions of global trade unfairly favour the MEDCs and the TNCs. Moves now being made by the World Trade Organisation to improve the conditions of trade need to be strengthened and speeded up. Actions include removing tariffs, subsidies and the cosy arrangements of powerful TNCs and trading blocs such as the EU and NAFTA.
- **Appropriate aid** Much of the aid extended by the MEDCs during the 20th century was in the form of loans. A significant proportion of that money was rightly spent on much-needed infrastructure projects, such as dams, power stations, roads, airports and telecommunications. Equally, large sums of money were misappropriated by corrupt governments and dictators. Unfortunately, loans attract interest and eventually have to be repaid. What too many LEDCs have discovered is that they are no longer able to service their debts. The knock-on effect is that countries enter a vicious circle of increasing debt, as new loans have to be taken out to repay existing ones. Desperately needed now

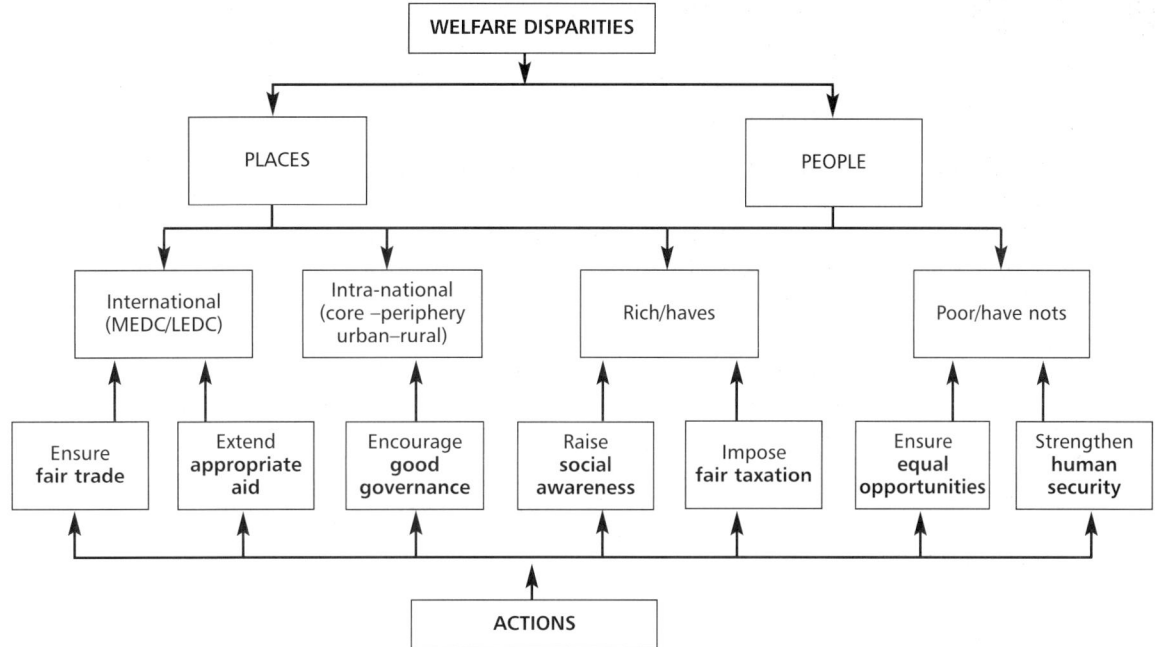

Figure 7.7 Reducing welfare disparities

are other forms of aid, particularly technical assistance and the transfer of technology. It would be better still for MEDCs to cancel the present debts and wipe the slate clean.

- **Good governance** This is needed if the disparities within a country are to be reduced. Basically, it requires (a) recognising those disparities, (b) understanding their causes and (c) taking appropriate remedial action. The last of these may often require action of either the 'stick and carrot' or the 'robbing Peter to pay Paul' varieties.

These three actions are aimed primarily at reducing spatial differences. The next four deal more with the disparities that exist between people (7.7).

- **Raise social awareness** What is needed here is education in the broadest sense; that is, making the more affluent people fully aware of the plight of the poor. At the same time, there is a need to instil a sense of responsibility to assist where and in whatever ways possible.
- **Fair taxation** No one likes taxes, but society does need a fair system whereby the financing of public services is based on ability to pay rather than use (a principle followed by micro-privatisation).
- **Equal opportunities** There are many factors involved here, but the most important are (a) ready access to education and the range of welfare services, and (b) freedom from discrimination on the basis of age, gender, class or ethnicity.
- **Protect human security** This is a more short-term action and requires protecting the security and sense of well-being of those who are less able to look after their own needs. The hope would be that once equal opportunities were assured, many such people would be able to fend for themselves. In the meantime, society needs to ensure that such people are adequately fed and housed, and are not marginalised.

With regard to the last of these actions, it is necessary to make reference once more to the horrific events of 11 September 2001 (**7.8**) and the global shock waves that have rippled out from them ever since.

There can be no doubting that those events have had a strongly negative impact on well-being and personal security at the whole range of scales from global to personal. At the time of writing (January 2002), we are only just beginning to wake up to the likely long-term consequences of those acts of terrorism. There is no doubting that the world order has been shaken. The global economy has sunk into recession and is unlikely to recover until some measure of confidence has been re-established. International terrorism has pushed the welfare of the world's needy down the global agenda. The global community needs to agree and implement a programme of appropriate action to deal with this destabilisation of the world order. The sooner this is done, the less the threat to our states of health and welfare – to yours, to mine and to that of others around the world.

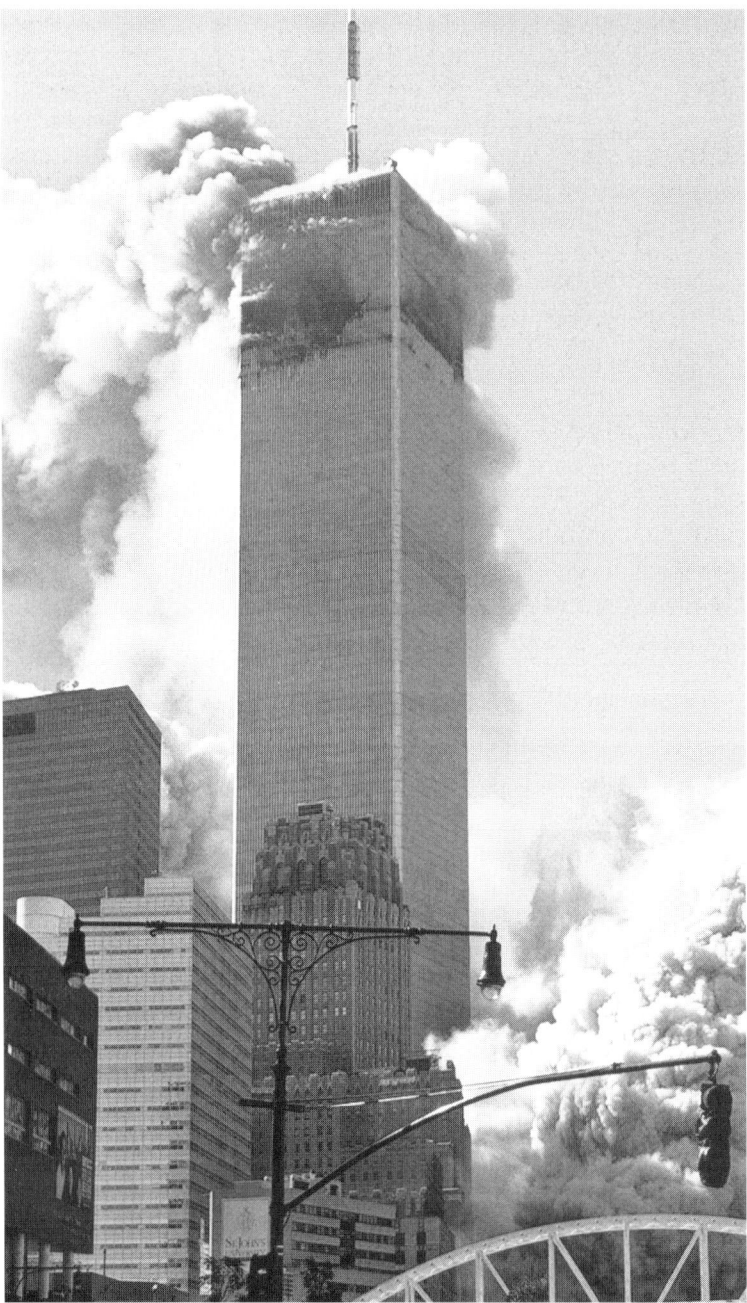

Figure 7.8 The destruction of the World Trade Center towers

Review

14 Identify ways in which the present conditions of global trade favour the MEDCs and TNCs.

15 Can you think of some 'stick and carrot' actions that have been taken by the UK government to reduce regional disparities?

16 Of the four bulleted actions to reduce disparities between groups of people, which would you nominate as the top priority? Give your reasons.

17 Explain why global insecurity is bad for welfare.

Enquiry

1 Research the link between ozone depletion and the three impacts shown in **7.2**.

2 Make an assessment of the relative state of health and welfare in your home county. This will involve:

- selecting and justifying a range of indicator measures
- obtaining relevant data from government (national and county) websites
- comparing your county against national norms
- producing a report that includes tables and diagrams to support your assessment.

Further reading and resources

Some book references include the following:

Andy Crump, *The A to Z of World Development* (New Internationalist Publications, 1998)

Anthony C. Gatrell, *Geographies of Health: an Introduction* (Blackwell, 2001)

Malcolm Harper, *Public Services through Private Enterprise* (Intermediate Technology Publications, 2000)

Eleanor Hill (ed.), *Development for Health* (Oxfam Publication, 1997)

Kelvin Jones and Graham Moon, *Health, Disease and Society* (Routledge & Kegan Paul, 1987)

David Smith, *Human Geography: a Welfare Approach* (Edward Arnold, 1977)

The latest edition of Philip's *Modern School Atlas* contains maps showing the global distributions of a wide range of health and welfare indicators.

Annual reports that provide up-to-date data and topical comment:

Philip's *Geographical Digest*

OECD, *Economic Surveys*

UNDP, *Human Development Report*

World Bank, *World Development Indicators*

World Health Organization, *The World Health Report*

Useful periodicals include *New Internationalist*, *New Scientist* and *People and the Planet*.

The Internet can be extremely helpful. All government, intergovernmental organisations and NGOs have their own websites, providing the very latest information. The following list summarises the websites used in the preparation of this book:

ActionAid: http://www.actionaid.org
AstraZeneca: http://www.astrazeneca.com
MSF: http://www.msf.org
Oxfam: http://www.oxfam.org
Planet 21: http://www.peopleandplanet.net
Shelter: http://www.shelter.org
UK statistics: http://www.statistics.gov.uk
UK government: http://www.ukonline
UK deprivation: http://www.detr.gov.uk

UK crime: http://www.homeoffice.gov.uk
UK health: http://www.doh.gov.uk
UK social services: http://www.dwp.gov.uk
UNAIDS: http://www.unaids.org
UNDP: http://www.undp.org
UNESCO: http://www.unesco.org
WHO: http://www.who.org
World Bank: http://www.worldbank.org